Your
Mental Health
Repair Manual

An Empowering, No-Nonsense Guide to Navigating Mental Health Care and Finding Treatments That Work for You

Pauline Lysak MD and Mark Roseman

Your Mental Health Repair Manual:
An Empowering, No-Nonsense Guide to Navigating Mental Health Care and Finding Treatments That Work for You

Copyright © 2019 by Pauline Lysak and Mark Roseman

All rights reserved. This book or any portion thereof may not be reproduced or used in any manner whatsoever without the express written permission of the publisher except for the use of brief quotations in a book review.

First edition: November 2019

ISBN: 978-1-9991495-4-3 (paperback)
ISBN: 978-1-9991495-5-0 (ebook)

Late Afternoon Press
Victoria, BC, Canada
lateaft.com

Edited by Peggy Herring
Cover design by Hina Shakti

To contact the authors
visit mhnav.com

The information in this book is not intended as a substitute for the medical advice of physicians. It is general and intended to better inform readers of their health care. Consult a physician for matters relating to your health and any symptoms that may require diagnosis or medical attention.

For all the patients we've had the privilege of working with—our greatest teachers.

Contents

Contents	v
Preface	vii
1. Introduction	1

Part I: A Primer on Mental Illness

2. What Is Mental Illness?	9
3. Diagnosing Mental Illness	15
4. The Mental Health System	21

Part II: Navigating Your Care

5. Taking an Active Role	29
6. Get Prepared	35
7. Family and Friends	39
8. Working With Your Family Doctor	43
9. Describing Your Symptoms	55
10. Working the Waiting List	61
11. Mental Health Interviews	67
12. Difficult Encounters	75

13. Paging Dr. Google	81
14. Your Living Treatment Plan	89
15. Using Your Plan	99

Part III: Treatments

16. So Many Choices!	111
17. Just Enough Neuroscience	115
18. Physical Illness	121
19. Lab Investigations	127
20. Lifestyle Factors	133
21. Vitamins and Supplements	143
22. Talk Therapy	151
23. Finding a Therapist	159
24. The Role of Medications	167
25. Antidepressants	177
26. Other Medications	191
27. Medication Side Effects	201
28. Evolving Your Medication Regime	211
29. Looking Ahead	221

Appendices

A. Internet Resources	227
B. Talk Therapies	231
C. Medications	239
Notes	259
Index	273
Acknowledgements	281
About the Authors	283

Preface

You know the mental health system is screwed up when you need a book to help you find decent care.

Awareness campaigns make it seem so easy. All will be better if you talk to someone about your mental health concerns. Doesn't that imply that if you do ask for help, you do talk, that you'll actually get some help? Just take that first step, and the mental health system will take care of you.

If you're reading this, chances are you haven't found the help you've been searching for. You may be looking for your own care or you may be supporting a family member or friend. You may even be a healthcare worker trying to help your patient or client. You've talked. You've asked. Still no help. All is definitely not better.

Your expectation of finding compassionate or humane care has faded. And confidence that someone will be there to take charge of your care? Please. At this point, you may be even more dejected, hopeless, lost, frustrated, and confused than when you started.

You're not alone in feeling this way. The lofty assurances that you just need to ask for help don't match the reality of mental health care.

Too Many Questions, Not Enough Answers

Most people find mental illness and its treatment mysterious. Few know what good care even looks like. That's where this book comes in. We'll pull back the curtain, put an end to the mystery, and explain what good mental health care is all about. With this insight, you'll be able to find better care.

Here's a typical path through the system. Your mental health is impacting your education, work, self-care, or family relationships. Like many people, you go to your family doctor for help. (If you're helping someone else, encouraging them to talk to their family doctor is also common.)

Your life, which seems to be falling apart, can't be fixed in the average 5- to 15-minute family doctor's appointment. Instead, your doctor prescribes an antidepressant and suggests some lifestyle changes, maybe provides a list of counsellors, the names of a few books or websites, and the local crisis line number. They might promise a referral to a psychiatrist. But don't get your hopes up, because the waiting list is six months long.

You leave your doctor's office and try to process what happened. If you're struggling to function, how are you supposed to wait around for half a year? And hope that the person you see can fix everything? You're confused and skeptical that a pill will help and overwhelmed just thinking about counselling. What do you do now?

Instead of a family doctor, you might start with a counsellor, psychologist, or another mental health professional. They might give you different options, but the gist of their response is pretty much the same.

If you had questions before, you still need answers to most of them:

- What's wrong with you?
- How are you supposed to know what kind of help you need?
- What are the treatment options? Why so many?
- How do you choose? What if you choose wrong?
- Why can't someone just tell you what to do?
- Where should you go? Who can help you?
- Why so many different opinions about what you should do?
- Will you end up stuck, going in circles, and not improving?

And that's if things go well. Some people who seek help are cut off and can't even share their concerns. Patients have told us that professionals answered their questions with, "there's nothing wrong with you," or "suck it up," or "I gave you a pill, what else do you want from me?"

You Can Do Better!

No large piles of money or quick fixes will address the structural flaws in the mental health system. When patients, their supports, and their healthcare providers don't know where to turn, it's a problem. When some family doctors recommend you Google local psychiatrists and cold call their offices to find one taking new patients, it's a problem. While stigma around mental illness is also a problem, for millions whose mental illness dramatically affects their life, being aware of their illness is not their problem. Finding help is their problem.

As a result, making the most of the help you do receive is critical. You're certainly willing to put the effort in. You want to be informed and involved. But it's hard when you receive partial and conflicting information. You're trying to get a sense of what's going on and how to move forward. You need a foundation to make sense of your options, and it's not there.

We can't magically change the system to deliver instant, top-notch care to everyone for every ailment. We can show you how to make the best use of the system we do have. And in mental health, there are many things you can do to dramatically improve care. These aren't big secrets. But a fragmented mental health system makes them very hard to find. We'll help you bring it all together to produce these results:

- You'll better understand your illness and its treatments.
- You'll help your health providers deliver better care.
- You'll proactively contribute to your treatment plan and care.
- You'll avoid unnecessary delays and wasting time.
- You'll stop feeling so confused and hopeless.
- Ultimately, you'll have a better chance at becoming well more quickly.

And in the immortal words of author Douglas Adams, *don't panic!* You won't need to read this entire book cover-to-cover. We've made it easy to find what you need and skip parts you may not need now. You can learn the essentials or go deeper on some topics. We'll explain more in the first chapter.

Empowerment Is Key

One of us (Pauline) is a psychiatrist who has been practicing for about fifteen years, spanning three Canadian provinces (Ontario, Alberta, and British Columbia) and various practice settings (public and private hospitals, outpatient mental health clinics, working directly with family doctors, and private practice). The other (Mark) has run Pauline's front office for several years. Besides (or despite) working together every day, we're also married.

Firsthand we've seen countless patients who had to wait months or years to receive care. All the while, their quality of life deteriorated. We've seen waiting lists grow, options for care disappear, and fewer psychiatrists available to help more patients. We've had to tell people who could no longer hold a job or keep their family together that we couldn't help them. We've seen newly pregnant women, worried about antidepressants in pregnancy, told to wait six months or longer for an appointment.

We've also heard from many people who waited a year or more to see a specialist. They were seen only once, too briefly to even tell their story, then given the wrong diagnosis or treatment. They were sometimes told what medication to take, unaware of the benefits, risks, or the existence of alternatives. Recommendations didn't help? Get back in line.

We've seen strain on the system, not only from a lack of resources. Sometimes resources were used inappropriately or unwisely. People who shouldn't have been sent to a psychiatrist were. People who should have weren't. Either someone thought it wasn't needed or nobody was available. We've seen many gaps in the system where people get stuck.

We've also seen countless missed opportunities. Simple actions not taken early on. Mistakes that could have been avoided. Well-meaning health professionals who could have done a few things differently but didn't have the time, expertise, or resources to provide better care.

We've also seen so many intelligent, capable, and resourceful people—who also happen to have a mental illness—unable to help themselves. Not because there's nothing they could have done, but because they couldn't easily find the information they needed. Most people, along with family and friends, are more than willing to put in some work if it helps and they have the skills. A modest investment in education is all it takes.

Who This Book Is For

Mental health uniquely affects each person. You may have the same mental health diagnosis as someone else, but your experience might be very different. Couple that with the fact that there are hundreds of mental health diagnoses. This makes it difficult to provide advice for everyone.

Illness-Inclusive

This book doesn't focus on a specific mental illness or diagnosis. While various forms of depression and anxiety are more common, the main issue—why you're not finding the care you need and not feeling better—is the same regardless of the diagnosis. So are the solutions to the problem. In terms of age, while some of what we discuss may benefit mature teens or parents of children with mental illness, this book deals with adult mental illness.

Moderate Severity

This book is geared toward people whose mental illness significantly interferes with one or more areas of their life but isn't completely debilitating. In severe illness, treatment options may be more limited, and people may not have the skills or motivation needed to help. They may not appreciate the impact of their illness, or even that they have an illness.

Instead, this book is for people who have an illness of mild to moderate severity. Hopefully, this includes you. If so, you appreciate the impact your illness is having on yourself and those around you. Though you may need help, you're able to continue in some capacity with several or even most basic activities, e.g., hygiene, getting out of the home, taking care of kids, shopping for groceries, and possibly working or going to school. You can have sensible interactions and conversations with others, though these may be limited. Most people seeking mental health care fit this profile.

High Functioning

You might worry that some days you're not as sharp as before. You can finish basic tasks, but they may be more difficult. You may have less energy or motivation, forget things more often if you don't write them down, or need to read things a few times before they stick. You may have more difficulty concentrating, trouble finding the right words to use, or you may become quickly frustrated.

Can you still take an active role in your treatment? Yes. Many people with mental illness experience similar cognitive difficulties. These aren't the same as you'd see in dementia. These challenges won't keep you from taking the meaningful steps to improve your mental health care that we'll cover in this book. You'll also find these symptoms usually improve as your underlying illness improves.

Friends and Family

Many people with mental illness are fortunate to have people in their life who support them. If you're one of those supporters, this book is for you, too. You will better appreciate what those close to you are experiencing. You'll learn how to work the system to better advocate for them. You'll also be better able to help them as they go to appointments, work with treatment providers, or experience setbacks. *Mental health is truly a team sport.*

In return, we beg your indulgence on one matter. We've chosen to write as if we're directly addressing people who require help with their mental health. We do not want to exclude you, given the invaluable help you provide, but wanted to save you (and everyone else) from some horribly convoluted writing.

Healthcare Professionals

Many healthcare professionals will also benefit from this book. If you work in healthcare, you've seen how mental illness affects all areas of your patients' lives. You've advocated on their behalf, trying to find help for their mental illness, only to face bureaucratic roadblocks and frustration. You may have even borne the brunt of their confusion or suffering, spending more time with them than the mental health specialist they see.

This book will help you better support your patients. If you're a family doctor, psychiatric nurse, psychologist, social worker or other mental health provider, you'll find it a good review of many topics and an introduction to areas you're less familiar with. You may even find some new and updated information. You'll also gain a fresh appreciation for the decision-making processes of other mental health professionals you work with each day.

As noted above, for clarity, this book speaks directly to those experiencing mental health challenges. We're not ignoring you!

Location, Location, Location

Finally, a quick note about where you live. While our direct experience is in Canada, we're mindful of the very significant differences between health systems in various jurisdictions. We draw examples from Canada, the USA, the UK, and elsewhere. The bulk of the book applies equally to people from any location, even if some fine details vary.

(Speaking of location, American readers should note that spelling follows the Canadian variant, e.g., "behaviour" versus "behavior.")

Except for the minority with an excess of money or influence, most people run into difficulties obtaining the mental health care they need. The reasons may vary based on how health systems are organized, funded, or accessed. Problems include long waiting lists due to a shortage of specialists, inability to pay, or restrictions on what insurance companies will cover. You've still got to make the most of what you've got.

Besides, while health systems vary, mental illness and how it's treated is pretty much the same wherever you go.

Let's get started.

1

Introduction

You've been distressed for months. You're frequently missing work and have lost touch with friends. You're becoming more withdrawn and skeptical about the future.

You've finally worked up the nerve to talk to a professional. You hope they might have a solution. Whether right after the first appointment or months down the road, you've realized you're not only still unwell, but more confused, desperate, and angry. You've lost hope that there is a solution and don't know where to turn.

Far too many people have this experience, particularly those seeking help for mental health problems for the first time. The mental health system makes it difficult for people to get the help they need. It's hard enough finding the right person willing to spend the time to listen to your problems, let alone someone who is able to help you fix them. You may waste time trying treatments that make you worse instead of better and miss those solutions likely to help.

It doesn't have to be that way. Part of the problem is that nobody tells you what the process of getting better looks like when you have a mental illness. How long should it take? What do the treatments do? The information that's out there is often piecemeal and scattered. It rarely reflects the practical realities of finding care. How then can you even tell the difference between good care and bad care?

All you know is you're not getting better. And you don't know how to fix it.

Take Control

You may be on a lengthy waiting list to see a professional. You may be going in circles with one or more treatment providers who seem to be fresh out of new ideas. You may feel abandoned and not sure where to turn next. Being on a waiting list isn't care. Neither is hoping for inspiration to strike. You have an important choice to make.

You can continue passively doing things as you have been. You can periodically raise your mental health concerns with your family doctor or other professional, hoping for a different response. If you've been referred to a psychiatrist or mental health clinic, you can sit back and wait until you're seen there. Your doctors are the experts. If there was something else you should be doing, they would have told you to do it.

Or you can learn and empower yourself. Get the best possible care you can within the system. You can work with your family doctor or another provider to move forward instead of waiting. Sometimes, a gentle nudge in the right direction is all it takes. You can learn to play a more active and productive role in your own care.

In other words, you can help bridge the gap between the sad reality of the mental health system and the comprehensive care you need.

The Sad Reality of Mental Health Care

To improve your care, you need to first understand what isn't working. People talk about a *mental health system*. In reality, it's less a system and more an uncoordinated patchwork of independent entities.

A true system would behave like an organization, with clear roles, responsibilities, processes, and procedures assigned to each part. Most importantly, there would be a map that ties each piece into an integrated whole. Despite the size and bureaucracy of many organizations that provide mental health care, groups inside and outside organizations rarely coordinate smoothly. Patients don't interact with a unified, coherent system.

Instead, providers move in different directions. Each sees itself in isolation, doing what they think they should be doing. There's no clear global accountability for results.

How can this affect you? After only a short time, if you're like most people, you'll find

- multiple, confusing entry points to access care;
- care not provided by the most appropriate providers;
- treatments often unhelpful or worse;

- standard of care for treatments often not met;
- poor communication between providers; and
- no progress tracking, resulting in being lost or stuck

To put it more simply, no one person is responsible for ensuring you get the care you actually need.

Comprehensive Care

If you want to do things differently, it helps to know what you're trying to accomplish. Even if you're taking on some of the work yourself, try to picture what a sensible patient-centred mental health care system would look like:

1. You'd know where to go to ask for help, and if that wasn't the right place, you'd quickly find your way to the right place.
2. You'd be properly diagnosed by a trained professional within a reasonable timeframe (i.e., days or weeks).
3. You'd know the plan to treat your illness, and you'd regularly check to make sure the plan is working. If not, the plan changes.
4. You'd involve the right professionals or resources as needed. All members of your care team would communicate with you and one another. Everyone shares the same view of your overall treatment plan, even if each person is responsible for only a particular part.
5. Nothing would be missed. If you became stuck or lost, you'd get back on track. All treatment would be appropriate to your needs.

We refer to this as *comprehensive care,* where all the necessary pieces are accounted for as part of a unified whole.

The Plan

What does taking a more active role in your treatment look like? It doesn't mean you're going to replace your doctors or other treatment providers—far from it. You're going to learn to work with them, even to do some things they can't. Together, as a team, you can get closer to achieving comprehensive mental health care.

To accomplish this, we'll help you do several things:

1. *Demystify mental illness.* A basic understanding of mental illness is the starting point. We'll try to clear up some common misconceptions and bring to light the most salient aspects of mental illness.

2. *Understand the mental health system.* Understanding some of the key pieces, the priorities, and the failures in the system will help you make the most of it and avoid frustration.

3. *Communicate.* You'll learn how to benefit from interviews with mental health providers, ensuring treatment decisions are based on the most accurate, important, and relevant information.

4. *Engage with professionals.* You'll learn how to access and productively work with a variety of treatment providers, not only counsellors, psychologists, and psychiatrists, but especially family doctors.

5. *Understand treatment options.* Knowing what different options are available and how they work allows you to suggest alternatives and maximize the effect of recommended treatments.

6. *Manage treatment.* Instructions, ideas, and opinions may come at you from many directions. Capturing them, organizing them, and sharing them with everyone involved can help increase collaboration, avoid missing essential steps, track progress, and speed up the entire process. We'll describe a tool called a *living treatment plan* that can help you with exactly that.

We didn't say this would be easy. You will have to learn a few things, but in a very focused and directed way. On the plus side, while mental health professionals have to learn a lot of things to help a lot of people, you will only need to learn enough to help you. And while all this research, communicating, and managing will take a bit of time, you're only doing it for one person.

Using This Book

This book is divided into three parts:

1. *A Primer on Mental Illness.* The first part will quickly run through the basics of mental illness. What is a mental illness? What causes it? How is one person's mental illness different from someone else's? How is a mental illness diagnosed? You'll also get a very high-level picture of the mental health system, the people in it, and some of its challenges. Depending on what you know to start with, you may want to quickly skim through this part.

2. *Navigating Your Care.* The second part will help you take a more active role in your own treatment. This is the core of the book. You'll learn what to expect, the questions to ask, and the many things you can do to make the whole process work to your advantage. You'll learn to

work and communicate effectively with doctors and others, helping them, and helping you. We'll touch on waiting lists, interviews, finding reliable health information, and keeping track of the big picture in a living treatment plan. This part will teach you what you need to become a full partner in your own treatment.

3. *Treatments.* Finally, the last part will introduce you to the wide range of treatments that can help with your mental illness. Yes, we'll talk about medications and therapy. You'll learn what antidepressants do and what makes one different from another. You'll learn about different psychotherapies, what they're used for, and how to find the right provider. You'll also learn about many other things that can improve or worsen your mental health: vitamins, supplements, exercise, caffeine, cannabis, and diet, to name just a few. There's a lot here, so you'll probably focus on only one or two parts at a time. It's the place to go when looking for ideas to bring forward or learning about treatments others suggest.

Each chapter is broken up into small sections, which should make it easier to skim over some parts and spend more time on other portions that you feel better suit your needs. To the extent possible, we've tried to minimize situations where you need to have a good understanding of the material in an earlier chapter to make sense of later material.

> Throughout the book, you'll find pockets of extra information that go into a bit more detail or help provide a deeper understanding of a topic. You'll be able to spot them because they're set off a bit from the rest of the book. This paragraph is an example of how they are formatted. These are optional. You can skip them entirely and you won't be missing anything critical that you'll need later.

You'll also find footnoted material collected at the end of the book. It will often point you to various articles, books, or websites that delve much further into a very specific topic. These include research on the effectiveness of different treatments.

Crucial Warning

We cannot emphasize enough how important it is for you to make changes to your medical or mental health treatment only in conjunction with your family doctor or other mental health professional.

We firmly believe in taking an interest in and accepting responsibility for your own healthcare. But you also should respect that you don't have the years of education and experience, or the perspective of trained professionals who have devoted their careers to this.

Mental illness can sometimes look simple, but it's not. For example, there's a big difference between feeling down and having clinical depression. Your brain is a complicated organ, intimately tied in with other body systems in a complex feedback loop. Making treatment decisions has consequences for your mental and physical health. Your doctor, in particular, has the background and training to anticipate and recognize those consequences.

While you will learn a lot about some of the causes and treatments of mental illness in this book, it only just scratches the surface. It's not a substitute for the expertise and judgment of professionals. Remember that mental illness can sometimes impair your judgment or cognition. Discuss, debate, challenge, agree, or disagree, but *never make actual changes on your own*.

The Payoff

All the effort you put into this will pay off. You'll be able to collaboratively come up with an effective treatment plan for your mental health concerns. You'll feel better faster. You'll get your life back more quickly. If you're on a waiting list to see a psychiatrist, your family doctor would like nothing more than to cancel the referral because it's no longer needed. The psychiatrist and the other people on their waiting list probably wouldn't mind either.

Even if you don't find a perfect solution, you'll certainly be further ahead than when you started. And knowing what hasn't worked will be valuable information to help the next professional you see find the right treatment for you. You'll also be a lot better informed and able to actively collaborate with your treatment providers.

Part I

A Primer on Mental Illness

2

What Is Mental Illness?

Over the next three chapters, we'll give you a crash course in mental illness. It will only cover the very basics but will be enough to make sense of the rest of this book as well as what mental health providers are telling you.

In the past, people knew little about mental illness. It was rarely discussed and a source of shame. People with mental illness were locked away in asylums, separated from society. Thankfully, the situation is better now. Most people today have some understanding of mental health and mental illness. They know that mental illness is not about character flaws or moral failures. It's a medical problem affecting people from all walks of life.

When it comes to getting more specific, it's challenging. Mental illness is vague in a way that a heart attack or diabetes isn't. As well, there are still some pretty big misconceptions out there. Let's fix that.

A Working Definition

Let's start with what *mental illness* means. Here's one definition:[1]

> *Mental illness refers to a wide range of mental health conditions—disorders that affect your mood, thinking, and behaviour…*
>
> *Many people have mental health concerns from time to time. But a mental health concern becomes a mental illness when ongoing signs and symptoms cause frequent stress and affect your ability to function.*

People use the term *physical illness* to cover a myriad of conditions such as appendicitis, a fractured hip, or breast cancer. In the same way, mental illness refers to a collection of more specific conditions such as obsessive-compulsive disorder or bulimia nervosa.

Everyone has times when they are sad, worried, or overwhelmed. Having ups and downs is normal. It's the frequency, duration and severity of symptoms that separate mental illness from everyday experience. Let's say you're diagnosed with clinical depression. A friend might try to help, telling you that they were depressed once. They had a good cry, went for a run, and all was good again. What they're describing is everyday life, not mental illness.

What Are the Different Types of Mental Illnesses?

Just as there are many physical illnesses, there are many mental illnesses too. In fact, there are around 200, depending on exactly how you count them. Table 2.1 lists the main categories of mental illness, and, in parentheses, the number of illnesses in each category. Most of these are then classified by subtype, specifier, features, or severity. Additionally, more than 40% of people who have a mental illness have two or more diagnoses at the same time. The illnesses are then said to be *comorbid*.[2]

Table 2.1: Categories of mental illnesses and disorders.

schizophrenia spectrum, psychotic (12)	depressive (8)
obsessive-compulsive and related (9)	anxiety (11)
trauma- and stressor-related (7)	dissociative (5)
neurodevelopmental (20)	elimination (4)
somatic symptom and related (7)	sleep-wake (18)
disruptive, impulse-control, conduct (7)	sexual dysfunctions (10)
substance-related and addictive (41)	gender dysphoria (3)
bipolar and related (7)	neurocognitive (18)
feeding and eating (8)	personality (13)
medication-induced movement, other	paraphilic (10)
adverse effects of medication (16)	other (4)

What Factors Lead to Mental Illness?

While the exact mechanisms are the subject of active research, most aren't well understood. The majority of experts think that many factors contribute to mental illness. This broad view is usually referred to as the *biopsychosocial model*. It says that biological factors (e.g., neurotransmitters, genetics) are part of the story, but not the whole story. Psychological (e.g., coping styles, attachment) and social factors (e.g., financial stress, culture) also play a role. They may all need to be addressed for optimal mental health.

One challenge for people seeking mental health care is finding care providers who address all parts of the biopsychosocial model. We'll return to this theme in various ways throughout the book.

Not everyone fully embraces the biopsychosocial model. Many agree with the model, but as a practical matter, provide only limited treatment options themselves. A psychiatrist who offers medication but recommends other providers for psychotherapy is an example. At a deeper level, some people reject the model altogether. They don't believe that all three components contribute to mental illness.

For example, some counsellors or laypeople don't think that biology has anything at all to do with mental health. At the extreme, they will tell you that since biology is not a factor in mental health, psychiatric medications don't treat anything, but are instead a government tool for social control.

At the other extreme are those who feel the only valid treatment for mental health is to address underlying biochemical deficiencies, genetics, inflammation, or effects of environmental contamination. Under a strictly biomedical model, mental illness is treated the same way an infection is treated. Bacteria causes the infection, and an antibiotic kills those bacteria.

Neither extreme reflects how mainstream medicine sees mental illness.

Episodic Versus Chronic Illness

It is important to distinguish between a single episode of mental illness that goes away after a short while and a mental illness that lasts longer.

Sometimes, you might experience mental illness for only a short time. This is often, but not always, in response to one or more events or stressors. It may go away on its own or with treatment. After that episode resolves, you may not have any further mental health concerns.

However, you may experience a chronic mental illness which lasts for a much longer period. It may wax and wane in intensity, but it's usually still there. You may have a recurrent illness, where you go through several distinct episodes of illness, broken up by periods where you're healthy.

Even a one-time episode of mental illness puts you at greater risk of having another episode in the future. For example, the odds of anyone having a major depressive episode in their lifetime are around 15%.

> If you've already had one episode, this jumps to 50% (and 70% after a second, and 90% after a third). Understanding the biopsychosocial factors that led to one episode may help reduce the risk of developing another.
>
> When we describe mental illness lasting a "short" time, remember it's not about regular ups and downs. Instead, it's far more intense and problematic. Most mental illness diagnoses require you to have experienced symptoms for a certain number of weeks or months.

Severity Matters

Severity is one aspect of mental illness that is often under appreciated.

There seems to be a stampede to diagnose any sign of mental turmoil as a mental illness. But for symptoms to represent a mental illness, they need to significantly impact a major area of your life (e.g., school, work, family, self-care). Two people may have the same diagnosis, but it doesn't mean the impact of that illness is the same. Consider these three individuals:

- Someone with social anxiety may be more nervous than the average person before giving a speech or when meeting someone new. But if this anxiety doesn't majorly impact their life, it's not mental illness.

- Faced with the same speech, someone with mild social anxiety disorder may be so nervous they need to psych themselves up for days beforehand. They may avoid it altogether. Still, they can hold down a job and keep relationships.

- That's very different from someone with severe social anxiety disorder. They may be unable to leave home or use the phone, to the point they can't look after themselves or their family, or go to work.

> It's more popular than ever to assign diagnoses. Around 19% of teenage boys are now diagnosed with ADHD (Attention-Deficit Hyperactivity Disorder), half before age six. Are people sicker now? Or, is there more pressure in many places to diagnose (and then treat) people? One recent study showed those under 19 in the USA were 72 times more likely to leave the hospital with a bipolar diagnosis than in the UK.[3]

One hundred per cent of people have room to improve their mental health. Many have specific mental health issues. But only approximately 18% have a diagnosable mental illness at any given time. And only about

4% of people have a severe mental illness. Most people with severe mental illness have a form of schizophrenia, severe bipolar, or severe depression. But if the impact is large enough, nearly any mental illness can be severe.[4]

This all has major public policy implications. It affects how scarce mental health funds are allocated. If "all mental health is equally important" do you invest in helping everyone "be the best they can be"? Or, do you invest in the vastly different needs of those with severe mental illness? To deliver the best mental health care, everyone can't be treated the same.

Severe Mental Illness

The more severe the illness, the bigger the impact on overall well-being and quality of life. Getting treatment for severe illness may mean the difference between a normal life and homelessness or worse. There are fewer effective treatment options as severity increases. Hardcore medications are needed, with specialists to administer and manage them. Awareness campaigns, peer counselling, and therapy programs may help some people with less severe illness. But these aren't very effective for those with severe illness.

> Helping yourself also assumes you know you're having a problem and that you want to fix it. One devastating symptom shared by many with severe mental illness is *anosognosia*. This is a belief that there's nothing wrong with you—so why would you want to seek treatment in the first place?
>
> This book won't help those with the most severe mental illness, who may not understand they have a problem, may have few treatment options, or who may be severely impacted by their illness. If dealing with reality is a major challenge, they may struggle to meaningfully participate in their own care. They're going to require more help from the system, which unfortunately isn't always there.

One Size Does Not Fit All

If there's one message we want you to take away, it's that mental illness is not a "one size fits all" term. Be very careful. What's right in one situation may be very wrong in another.

Keep this in mind when people give you advice based on their own experience with mental illness. It may be similar to what you're experiencing but could be very different. The solutions that worked for them may not be helpful for what you're facing. Whether we're talking about mental illness in general or even one illness, it's still a huge number of people. It's very easy to overgeneralize, merge very different subgroups, or abuse statistics.

Here are two claims about mental illness where more nuance is needed:

- *Medications aren't needed to treat mental health.* As you saw, the severity of mental health and mental illness can vary greatly. Many with mild mental health issues or mental illness may not need any treatment at all. For many with mild to moderate mental illness, treatment with medications may be a useful option. So might many other types of treatments, alone or in combination. However, as severity increases, the need for treatment increases, while options for effective non-pharmaceutical treatment decrease.

- *If you have a mental illness, you'll be committed to a hospital and treated against your will.* Actually, very few people are ever forced to stay in hospital or forcibly treated. This happens only in the most severe crisis situations, where there is a risk of imminent danger to self or others. The specifics of involuntary commitment and treatment legislation vary across jurisdictions. With too few inpatient psychiatry beds, the pressure is to help people outside of hospital, not vice versa.

Watch out for people making sweeping generalizations about mental illness. Remember, there are many different mental illnesses. Even two people sharing the same diagnosis may have completely different experiences.

Summary

- Mental illness is a blanket term for a very large number of individual illnesses, each varying greatly in how it affects individuals.
- About one in five people will experience a mental illness, which can have severe effects on their functioning, as well as on those around them.
- The biopsychosocial model reflects the view that mental illness is brought on by a mix of biological, psychological, and social factors, and its treatment may require intervention in one or more of these areas.
- With such variety in illnesses, symptoms, severity, and causes, there are no "one size fits all" solutions. Take care to avoid generalizations or assuming one person's experience applies to someone else.

3

Diagnosing Mental Illness

If your family doctor wants to know if you have an infection, they'll order a blood test. To check for a broken bone, they'll do an X-ray. For heart problems, maybe an electrocardiogram makes sense. What test can diagnose someone with major depression? With obsessive-compulsive disorder? Posttraumatic stress disorder?

Some people are surprised to find out that there are no laboratory tests to diagnose a mental illness. No blood tests, CT scans, or anything else. Instead, a diagnosis is based on your symptoms. You describe symptoms while giving your history and answering questions from your health provider. Their observations, and sometimes those of family and friends, also help establish the diagnosis.

With no tests to diagnose it, some people believe mental illness is not real. They are wrong. Mental illness is very real. Many physical illnesses are also diagnosed solely from their symptoms. Most syndromes (Wikipedia lists over 1,400) fit that category, e.g., irritable bowel syndrome or post-concussion syndrome. Other illnesses now have tests that didn't exist in the past. Genetic tests identify mutations associated with some illnesses, while advanced imaging can see brain changes characteristic of other ailments. Perhaps someday researchers will identify tests for specific mental illnesses.

What Defines a Specific Illness?

To make a diagnosis, your doctor evaluates your symptoms against a set of criteria for a certain illness. If the doctor feels you meet those criteria, then you have that illness. Think of it like taking a test that you'd rather not pass.

What do the criteria for a mental illness look like? Here's an example for binge-eating disorder. Note the specifics on duration and impact.

(A) Recurrent episodes of binge eating. An episode is characterized by both of the following:

1. Eating, in a discrete period of time (e.g., within any 2-hour period), an amount of food that is definitely larger than what most people would eat in a similar period of time under similar circumstances.
2. A sense of lack of control over eating during the episode (e.g., a feeling that one cannot stop eating or control what or how much one is eating).

(B) The binge-eating episodes are associated with three (or more) of the following:

1. Eating much more rapidly than normal.
2. Eating until feeling uncomfortably full.
3. Eating large amounts of food when not feeling physically hungry.
4. Eating alone because of feeling embarrassed by how much one is eating.
5. Feeling disgusted with oneself, depressed, or very guilty afterwards.
6. Sleep disturbance (difficulty falling or staying asleep, or restless, unsatisfying sleep).

(C) Marked distress regarding binge eating is present.

(D) The binge eating occurs, on average, at least once a week for 3 months.

(E) The binge eating is not associated with the recurrent use of inappropriate compensatory behaviour as in bulimia nervosa and does not occur exclusively during the course of bulimia nervosa or anorexia nervosa.

Who Defines Illnesses?

The criteria for every mental illness come from a thick book called the Diagnostic and Statistical Manual of Mental Disorders, Fifth Edition (DSM-5), published by the American Psychiatric Association. New versions are the product of years of meetings and debates by experts in all areas of mental health.

The DSM-5 reflects the current mainstream understanding of different mental illnesses. It highlights the clinically relevant symptoms that identify each illness and helps providers differentiate between them. It gives mental health professionals a common language to communicate with one another.

The DSM-5 has much more on each illness than just the list of criteria, including diagnostic features, prevalence, development, course, risk factors, culture- and gender-related issues, differential diagnosis, and comorbidity.

The DSM-5 is nicknamed the "bible" of psychiatry. But it was written by people, some with vested interests, and is not infallible. There are heated disagreements about issues large and small. How are illnesses categorized? How relevant are certain symptoms? What should or should not be considered a disorder? The DSM evolves over time, alongside the theory and practice of mental health care. Think of it as a guidebook and judge it by how well it helps guide people back to health.

Many people, for a variety of reasons, are skeptical of psychiatry. They believe that the mental health system medicalizes normal human emotion. They fear that every thought and feeling will eventually be evidence of some disease. These people ignore that symptoms have to significantly interfere with your life to suggest an illness. You certainly wouldn't choose to treat it otherwise.

Mental Illness Categories

You saw earlier that mental illnesses are organized into about 20 categories in the DSM-5. These categories can be convenient, but it's the specific illness that matters when you want to treat it. It's useful to talk about depressive disorders versus anxiety disorders, but a category isn't a diagnosis.

One category that generates a lot of confusion and misunderstanding is *personality disorders*. Personality disorders are diagnosed when people have significant and longstanding difficulty coping with life events. They have unhealthy or inflexible coping strategies that cause tension in relationships with others. Here are two examples:

> - Imagine you are someone who is very distressed by uncertainty. You may cope by trying to control everything around you. If this has a large enough impact on your life, you may be diagnosed with obsessive-compulsive personality disorder.
> - Imagine a friend tells you they are unavailable to have coffee with you. Most people would see this as a minor disappointment. But you might decide they cancelled because they hate you. As a result, you might feel abandoned and become so distressed you engage in self-harm such as cutting. These are hallmarks of borderline personality disorder, one of the most stigma-laden mental illnesses.
>
> Personality disorders are difficult to diagnose and often misdiagnosed. They're present even during long periods when mood, anxiety, etc. are not problematic. They tend to occur in direct response to life events. Other disorders are not always as strongly tied to life events. Providers need a thorough, long-term history to correctly diagnose a personality disorder.
>
> Personality disorders don't respond as well to some short-term treatments or medications used for other illnesses. At best, these temporarily reduce impulsive, unhealthy coping behaviours. Without specific therapy, people with personality disorders often bounce from one crisis to another without getting better. The hospital emergency room can get them past the crisis but isn't the right setting to treat people with personality disorders.

Can Anyone Diagnose a Mental Illness?

If diagnosis is as simple as using a checklist of criteria, can anyone do it? Can you diagnose yourself? Can you diagnose one of your relatives? Making an accurate mental health diagnosis is not that simple.

First, you'd need to be familiar with the hundreds of different disorders in the DSM-5. You'd need to know what symptoms to look for, how to identify them, and be able to rule out other diagnoses. It's too easy to focus on one or two things and miss many others. Having an incomplete picture of what's going on with someone is a recipe for misdiagnosis.

You may have identified all relevant symptoms and know the criteria. It's still a skill to know how to interpret those criteria—how severe the symptoms have to be, for example.

Many mental health symptoms can also be symptoms of other illnesses. That makes a general knowledge of medicine essential. Often, the first signs of a brain tumour are changes in behaviour. You don't want to quickly pass that off as some mild mental illness.

Making an accurate diagnosis requires substantial knowledge, skill, and experience. Being able to do it well is an art. It also explains why psychiatrists complete five or more years of theoretical and practical training after undergraduate and medical school. They are taught to diagnose and treat the full range of mental illnesses. Yes, your psychiatrist is a real doctor. At one time, they helped deliver babies, performed surgery, and did spinal taps.

People other than psychiatrists frequently diagnose and treat mental illness. Family doctors have comprehensive health knowledge including training in mental health. Psychologists may have more mental health training, though lack the medical background. Their diagnosis may come with the caveat that they can't exclude other physical illnesses.

If something seems unusual or if the standard treatment isn't working, they may recommend a psychiatrist. These are hints that something else may be going on, and getting a fresh look, including reviewing your diagnosis, may help.

You may have people in your life now who are telling you what's wrong with you or insisting that nothing is wrong. How much should you depend on what they say?

How Important Is a Specific Diagnosis?

Does the exact mental health diagnosis really matter that much?

If you have chest pain, you want to know whether it's from a heart attack, pneumonia, acid reflux, or a pulled muscle. You *really* want to know before someone decides to crack your chest open to perform surgery.

As with physical health, the same symptoms can suggest different illnesses. Someone with frequent suicidal thoughts may be suffering from a form of depression. They may have an entirely different illness such as borderline personality disorder. The two are treated very differently. Poor concentration may be a symptom of depression or anxiety. It could be due to attention-deficit hyperactivity disorder, low iron levels, or other things. Treating the wrong problem is not likely to be helpful. An antidepressant won't fix poor concentration due to ADHD. Cognitive behavioural therapy for anxiety will not address an iron deficiency.

To complicate matters, having two or more (comorbid) mental illnesses at the same time is common. Some of your symptoms may be explained by one illness and other symptoms by another. Sometimes there will be overlap. It's also common to have a mental illness with a comorbid physical illness. In fact, if you have certain physical illnesses, you have a much greater chance of also having some mental illnesses.

At the same time, it's easy to get too carried away with specific details. Will it really matter if a major depressive disorder is classified as severe versus moderate? Probably not. Don't get too worked up over it. Sometimes it makes sense to label your illness "Herbert," and get on with it!

As another example, say the criteria for an illness requires you to have six of twelve symptoms. You may only have five, but those five are causing you significant distress. Yes, you don't technically have the illness. But it also may not hurt to treat you as if you fully met the criteria. The same thinking applies when you may have all the symptoms, but one is not quite severe enough.

Sometimes patients with comorbid illnesses get hung up on their diagnoses a bit too much. They obsess about whether something they did was because of their anxiety or their ADHD. A diagnosis is just a tool, valuable only as long as it's useful in helping you become well.

Summary

- As with many physical illnesses, there are no laboratory investigations yet that definitively diagnose a mental illness.

- Each mental illness is defined by a set of specific criteria, but there are usually multiple ways to meet criteria for an illness; comorbid mental illnesses (more than one at a time) are also common.

- The DSM-5 defines the criteria and provides a great deal of additional information on each illness. Specific training and expertise are needed to interpret and apply this information.

- A mental illness is only diagnosed when symptoms are severe enough to have a significant impact on functioning.

4

The Mental Health System

In most places, mental health care functions as anything but a unified system. It's often seen as an unconnected and unevenly distributed collection of independent providers and services. There's no standard path through the system to follow. Getting lost or stuck is a widespread problem. You need to find the right resources to get the care you need.

To find your way, you need to know what the system looks like. What are the different pieces? Where do you find them? What can they provide? Where are the gaps in the system? Let's look at these in more detail.

Crisis? What Crisis?

The good news is that if your mental illness is severe enough or you're actively suicidal, it's usually possible to access some help, at least in the short term. This is often through emergency rooms or a short-term crisis service.

The bad news is, when it comes to quickly accessing mental health treatment, things usually have to be really bad to be considered bad enough.

You may be crying all the time, unable to get out of bed.

You may be so stressed that you're not able to work.

You may be so easily angered and unpredictable that your family is ready to walk out the door.

These horrible situations can ravage your life. But they may not be bad enough for you to receive urgent mental health care. Unfortunately, while millions of people may be suffering from mental illness impacting their employment, relationships, and personal well-being, most of them cannot promptly access specialized mental health care.

Squeezed in the Middle

You may think that the mental health system was not built for you, and you're right. On one extreme, you've got motivational books and speakers. They promote self-awareness, personal growth, and development. They're happy to exchange your money for a promise of an even better you. On the other extreme, you've got the hardcore psychiatric services. They deal with the most severe chronic mental illnesses or people who are in an urgent crisis.[1]

Where do you fit? Probably somewhere in between. You may not be in a life-threatening crisis now, but your illness is having a major impact on your life. You're not trying to be the absolute best version of yourself but want to get back to where you were before your symptoms started. Increasingly, it seems that if there isn't a quick and easy fix, you've got few places to turn. You're far less likely to see a psychiatrist or another mental health specialist. If you do, it will probably only be for a short time. Many systems can help if you're in crisis, but don't do as well once the immediate crisis passes.

Where Are Mental Illnesses Treated?

You've decided it's time to get help. Great! Now what? Your first question is likely to be "where do I go?" Table 4.1 suggests a few common answers.

Table 4.1: Some places where people seek mental health help.

family or friend	support group
school guidance counsellor	mental health association
crisis line	workplace human resources
clinical counsellor	library or bookstore
psychologist	priest or other religious figure
internet	hospital emergency room
spiritual elder	family doctor, psychiatrist, other MD

Treatment takes place in all kinds of settings. It can be at home, by yourself, going through a workbook. It can be at a peer support group held in a community centre basement. Many mental health professionals work in private offices, alone, with a few colleagues, or in a larger organization. You may be treated in a medical clinic or hospital.

So many people, places, and programs. Each plays a role in the overall mental health system. Each offers something different. What do you need? How do you choose?

It's hard to keep track of all the professionals in mental health. One common confusion is the difference between psychiatrists and psychologists.

A psychiatrist is a medical doctor. After the standard training for any doctor (undergraduate and medical school), they complete a five-year residency across different areas of mental health. Their practice can include a wide range of treatment options, including medications, psychotherapy, laboratory or imaging investigations, etc.

Psychologists typically have a master's degree or PhD in psychology or a related field. Their practices generally involve psychotherapy of some form.

Many psychiatrists and psychologists have specialized practices, either involving particular illnesses or particular treatments. We'll have a lot more to say throughout the book about other differences and the importance of seeking care from the full range of mental health professionals.

Can You Afford It?

For many people, the cost of mental health care whittles down their choices very quickly. Cost, access, and restrictions are always complicated. Services vary greatly depending on where you live. Government programs and insurance may have strict limits on what services they cover, how many, and who provides each service. They won't pay pricey psychiatrists to do psychotherapy if a counsellor can do it for less.

If medications become part of your treatment, you will have to pay for them. If you have private insurance, it may pay for some or all of them. Government plans may help some reduce the cost of medications.

If you're financially well off or have a job with great benefits, you can access a wide range of treatments, through family doctors, psychiatrists, psychologists, and counsellors. If you're less well off, you'll probably see a family doctor who will prescribe a low-cost antidepressant. If you're lucky, you'll participate in subsidized group education and therapy programs for a few months.

The Critical Role of Medical Doctors

We won't say that you should only see a medical doctor for your mental health. But we do think they should be one of the people you see. This is especially true if you've been struggling with mental health symptoms for a long time, or if your symptoms came on rapidly with no obvious cause.

Why see a medical doctor? Sure, they're the only ones who can prescribe medications such as antidepressants that are so much a part of modern-day treatment. But there's a far more important reason to see a doctor. Many mental health symptoms can be signs of physical illnesses—sometimes serious ones. Finding and treating these illnesses can improve your overall health. Treating the physical illness may also address your mental health concerns, sometimes very quickly.

You may never intend to take a mental health medication. That's fine, but make sure there's nothing physical going on. See a doctor.

Psychiatrists

When most people think about seeing a doctor for their mental health, they picture a psychiatrist. They specialize in feelings, behaviours, and thoughts.

Like other doctors, psychiatrists see people in different settings, such as the emergency room or an inpatient psychiatry ward in a hospital. However, most people are seen as outpatients, having short visits with a psychiatrist in a hospital, clinic, or office. Some psychiatrists care for people with many mental illnesses. Others may treat only some types of illnesses, and a few are very specialized, treating only a single illness.

Family Doctors

Most people go for mental health care to the same place they go for their other health needs: their family doctor's office.

Mental health is a standard part of every family doctor's training, and something they help with each day. Around 20% of family doctor appointments involve a mental health issue.[2] Multiple studies found that most people with a mental health disorder (one suggested as high as 85%) see *only* their family doctor. Many family doctors manage most cases of common mental illnesses such as depression and anxiety themselves. They're often more likely to recognize or test for physical problems. Often, family doctors need to assess and refer you before you can see a psychiatrist.

We will have a lot to say about the important role that family doctors play in the mental health system. Learning to work well with your family doctor is one of the best things you can do for your mental health.

Hurry Up and Wait

Frequently, by the time people ask for help, a lot of time has already passed. You want to get things moving now. You want help, a path forward. You'd like to see a plan and know how long it will take.

If you've been at this for a while, you know there is no plan. Instead, there's waiting. Let's say you were experiencing depression and saw your family doctor about it. Here are some delays you might face:

1. You wait days or weeks to see your family doctor. You spend months trying the medication they prescribe. It makes you physically ill from side effects, but your mood remains unchanged.
2. You spend months with a counsellor or in a community therapy group, but nothing changes.
3. You feel that your family doctor is sick of listening to you complain and has run out of ideas. You wait months before bringing up that you're still not coping. They refer you to a psychiatrist.
4. You wait months or longer for your appointment with the psychiatrist. They see you only once, for a total of 45 minutes. You then wait for your family doctor to receive the psychiatrist's report.
5. You spend weeks trying the new medication the psychiatrist recommended, which doesn't work. You wait even longer to be referred back to that same psychiatrist or a different one for another opinion.

All this and your symptoms are just as bad as when you started. Sadly, this is still better than being stuck, not knowing what to do next, and not having anyone to ask. Is this what mental health care should look like?

System Failures

We described the mental health system as an uncoordinated patchwork of independent service providers. Each one works in isolation according to its own priorities. This creates several problems for you:

- There are multiple entry points to access care. There's no way to know which is the most appropriate for your needs. Tellingly, most people working in the system are also frequently stumped.
- Transitions between care providers can be ad hoc or non-existent. If one can't help you, they may not send you to someone more appropriate. Some may not understand the value that other providers bring.
- You may be treated by people untrained in your actual problem. Patients are routinely misdiagnosed or receive different diagnoses from different providers. Treating the wrong illness will be unhelpful at best and may worsen your condition.
- Even with the right diagnosis, all recommended tests and treatments may not be provided. Communication between providers is limited. One provider may assume another has addressed specific issues.

- As more providers are added, care becomes more fragmented and poorly integrated. Treatments from different providers seem independent of one another and can even work at cross purposes.
- Nobody is tracking where you are on your journey from illness to wellness. Intuitively, you understand that you're not making progress. But without knowing what the treatment process should look like, you can't form expectations to measure your progress against.

Consequences

There are many different kinds of mental health providers to choose from who offer a dizzying array of services. Seeing a provider who is unable to help you is common. Without someone to guide you, it's too easy to get lost in the system. Your care could stall altogether.

Thankfully, you can do better.

Summary

- Mental illness is treated by a wide range of professionals in a variety of settings.
- Psychiatrists and family doctors play an important role, as many symptoms of mental illness can be symptoms of an underlying physical illness.
- Access to mental health care can be difficult, with a limited number of professionals available, and many insurance and other financial barriers. Much of this is related to how mental health is prioritized.
- The idea of mental health as a system is misleading. Most providers are independent, there are multiple paths through the system, and people often don't see providers appropriate for their needs. People often get lost or stuck and don't receive the treatment they need.

Part II

Navigating Your Care

5

Taking an Active Role

The first part of this book explains how difficult it can be to find the mental health care you need in a timely manner. In this second part, you'll learn what you can do about it. You'll discover practical tools, strategies, tips, and techniques to avoid the pitfalls of the system. You'll create new opportunities and learn to maximize each one.

Some approaches we'll describe were impossible ten years ago. Others were once heretical to the medical establishment. Maybe if you're the kind of person who has already researched your symptoms and treatments, what you learn here will be a natural progression. However, if you've instead assumed a more traditional or passive role in your health care, what you learn may represent a far greater change.

We'll begin by introducing the concept of *patient navigation*, which is critical to getting the best mental health care possible.

Managing the Big Picture

Simple problems often have simple solutions, even in a field as complex as medicine. You develop an infection, you see your family doctor. They order a blood test that confirms an elevated white blood cell count. They prescribe an antibiotic that you take for several days. If you're better after that, you're all done.

Mental illness is rarely that simple. Diagnosis is difficult, sometimes taking months or years. Finding the right treatment takes more time and much trial and error. You might need monitoring and ongoing adjustments to your treatment. This long-term or chronic approach to care is very different than dealing with a simple infection.

Managing chronic illness is not easy. There are many moving pieces. Often, certain tasks (and people!) fall through the cracks. One doctor doesn't order a test because they assume another doctor already did. The second assumes the first ordered it. Both wait on the test results before proceeding. If you cancel an appointment, does someone ensure it's rescheduled? Does anyone check that a treatment is working, one, two, or six months later? If symptoms worsen, is that brought to the right person's attention and dealt with promptly? Or, more typically, are problems forgotten until you remember to ask at your appointment—six months later?

In the past, your family doctor kept an eye on this process. They'd notice if things went south, pick up the pieces, and get everything back on track. They can't do this anymore. It takes all their attention to focus on the complex problems in front of them right now. Medicine today is more complicated, and doctors can't keep up. You need new ways to monitor your overall progress.

Mental illness may be the most challenging chronic illness to manage. It can involve many professionals in very different fields. People with the same diagnosis and symptoms can all react very differently to the same treatment. While the science behind mental health is progressing, it's decades behind other areas of medicine.

No one can fix the problem by just throwing more money at it. Even if the money were there—which it isn't—to add more doctors, counsellors, etc., the complexity remains. Improving your mental health care needs a new way of thinking.

Patient Navigators

There is a helpful model in some other areas of medicine called *patient navigation*. We'll show you how it's used in cancer care, and then see how it could be adapted to mental health.

In cancer care, many professionals work together to help each patient. These include family doctors, medical oncologists, radiation oncologists, surgeons, nurses, pharmacists, dieticians, social workers, and others. Each has a role to play that depends on what happens when patients see others in the system. If tests are delayed or lost, or if patients don't see the right doctors at the right time, it can mean the difference between life and death.

Cancer treatment is complex, confusing, and stressful. To help manage this, dedicated cancer centres are created where the many different care providers can work closely together. Each patient is assigned a *patient navigator*. Their only job is to ensure that everything that patient needs gets done, and nothing falls through the cracks. They know the system, the players, and what happens at what time during treatment. They'll book appointments and tests, and make sure the results get to the right people. They'll help you with any questions, chasing down answers on your behalf.

Patient navigation is not entirely new. It has existed informally for decades. People often bring family members and friends to medical appointments or case conferences. They discuss their care with them, ask for advice, and entrust them with day-to-day organization involving their care. Family and friends may ask other medical people they know for help from time to time. Yet, having a dedicated person responsible for all this is a recent phenomenon.

Even more recent are third-party, privately-paid patient navigators. They are neither hired by the healthcare institution, nor are they friends or family. Instead, you or your family hire them the same way you'd hire a lawyer or accountant.[1] This is an area of the healthcare industry still in its infancy but poised for growth.[2]

Could mental health use this model? It's obvious that the current fragmented and short-term approach to care is failing many people. But is anyone in the system ready to pay for patient navigators? Definitely not.

So, is that the end of the story? We believe the answer to that question is a clear no. As we turn again to informal and unpaid patient navigation, keep in mind the roles and responsibilities of dedicated patient navigators. Can family, friends, and patients themselves accomplish the same things? Most definitely, particularly when it comes to the management and process of mental health care. These are shaky aspects of the system now, and ripe for improvement.

As we've said before, this is not something that applies to all patients or all areas of mental health care. If you're having a major psychotic episode or extreme depression, you may not be able to manage much of your care. However, if you're one of the high-functioning majority with mild to moderate mental illness, you've got the skills and capabilities. Assisting with the management of your care is entirely within reach.

Changing Attitudes and Opportunities

The capacity for patients to help with management, coordination, and advocacy in their own mental health is new. In the past, doctors held all the medical knowledge, gathered from their long training and the dusty books and journals on their shelves. Anyone else seeking such knowledge would trek to a medical library and spend hours in the stacks trying to decipher arcane tomes of technical jargon. From that, they might gain a basic understanding of a topic. Now, this seems archaic.

Today, we have an overabundance of information available to anyone. Much of it doesn't presume formal medical training, though a lot of it is also of dubious quality. The internet has levelled the playing field. Even many doctors find "Dr. Google" faster than digging up that one journal article in their overflowing filing cabinets.

Attitudes toward patient involvement in medical care are also—slowly—changing. In the past, doctors' proclamations were gospel. Today, patients download their own lab results. They bring their own research and treatment alternatives to appointments. They expect to learn about the relative merits of different options and participate in treatment decisions. Medical students today learn the soft skills of collaborative problem solving and team-based care.

Modern mental health care offers many opportunities for patients to contribute and play a more active role in their care. For example, measuring symptoms and severity is time-consuming. Much of it is based on subjective self-reporting. Patients can track many of these at home without their doctor's direct involvement. A doctor asking the same set of questions each appointment is often a poor use of limited time. When it comes to learning about and engaging in discussions about treatment, the complexity of the underlying science doesn't need to be an obstacle. Patients can use simpler mental models without having advanced neuroscience degrees.

Active Collaboration

You should have options beyond the traditional paternalistic model of medical care where doctors always know best and patients don't question them. Why shouldn't you be an active member of your treatment team, making decisions in collaboration with your care providers?

For this to work, both patients and providers must recognize what each brings to the table, including their limitations. Doctors have broad medical knowledge, experience treating mental illness, access to medical tests, and resources. They know the many causes of symptoms and consequences of treatments. You have first-hand knowledge of your own experiences. You can learn about your illness, track its progress, and manage your day-to-day care. You can weigh the benefits and risks of different treatments. You have far more time to spend on your own care than your doctor.

Not everyone can or wants to take on these responsibilities. But, in our experience, countless people are able and very willing.

Better care can be a reality. What it takes is learning a specific set of skills and how to apply them. By doing so, you help not just yourself, but the whole system, in effect adding much-needed capacity, without asking for the impossible: more investment of public funds.

Let's now turn to the skills you'll need.

> ### Summary
> - Chronic illnesses, including mental illnesses, are increasingly difficult to manage. It's more complicated as care evolves over time and when multiple treatment providers are involved.
> - Patient navigators help organize care for chronic illnesses such as cancer. They see the big picture, coordinate providers, and ensure tests and follow-up are arranged. They prevent patients from getting lost or stuck in the system.
> - Medicine has evolved from a model where only doctors had access to medical knowledge and made decisions. Now, patients expect to be involved in decision making and have access to an unprecedented amount of medical research.
> - Active collaboration refers to patients and their supports taking on more responsibilities for navigation and tracking tasks. It means working with doctors and other care providers as a team to provide a better level of care.

6

Get Prepared

Take a deep breath. You're about to start a journey that will transform you into a better-educated and more successful patient. You'll learn what sort of mental health care you need and how to get it. Just as a long road trip requires planning in order to avoid problems, this journey will also go smoother with some preparation.

This book will teach you a variety of new skills. But you're not starting from scratch. You're already familiar with many of the tools that will help you along the way. Part of your journey will entail knowing which tools to bring along as well as which ones to leave behind, including perhaps any pre-existing expectations of how health care should work.

Basic Tools of the Trade

Lots of information is going to be thrown at you, both by us and by your care providers. Do you have a photographic memory and the ability to absorb everything you hear? If not, get yourself a notebook, always carry it, and make a habit of using it. There's a reason most people take notes when learning something new. Writing information down helps you absorb it at the time and provides a reminder later. This is doubly important as lapses in memory are common in mental illnesses.

We'll offer suggestions for organizing your thoughts, questions, and aspects of your treatment plan. For now, think of it as taking notes in school. Are you one for stickers, post-its, multicolour highlighters, or even a fancy pen? If so, treat yourself to a trip to your favourite office supply store. Is your smartphone, tablet, or laptop easier, faster, and more convenient than a paper notebook? Go with what works for you.

If you have copies of existing health records, mental health or otherwise, keep them where you can easily get at them. If your mental health struggles have been going on for a while, put together a brief timeline of events. It should include treatments you've already tried. We'll talk much more about this in the chapter titled *Your Living Treatment Plan*.

Some people think they have a single definitive medical record out there, containing their complete medical history. In reality, there is no one true medical record. Instead, you've got bits and pieces of partial information, perhaps inconsistent and out of date, spread across the filing cabinets and servers of your past and present treatment providers. Nobody has a complete picture. What little coordination exists is haphazard at best.

You're going to need to do some research about mental illness, treatments, and providers. These days, much of that will require using the internet. Access to a smartphone, tablet, or computer is necessary. Libraries are great if you don't have your own device. If you're not familiar with the technology, it shouldn't be too hard to find someone to help.

Reset Your Expectations

One of the best things you can do is rid yourself of any expectation about how mental health care should work. Yes, it should be easy to connect with someone who can quickly get you the help you need. If you're reading this book, it's a given that reality fell short of your expectations. You'll need to do many things that you never expected to do. Some things may be uncomfortable.

- Others won't always direct you to the care you need. Sometimes you'll need to both find opportunities for care and push to access them.
- Professionals won't always give you details or answer your questions. You'll need to find information on your own.
- You might expect people to help you or direct you to someone who can. Instead, you'll have people simply saying no or telling you there's nothing they—or anyone—can do. Get used to hearing no but pushing on despite that.
- You can't wait passively and trust that someone will take care of you. You must be active and advocate for yourself.

- You might expect a quick or obvious solution to your mental health issues. You'll need to learn patience and understand that finding a solution may take time. Changing direction along the way is an unavoidable part of the process.
- Most people become frustrated by the bureaucracy and inefficiency in the mental health system. Little wonder that most patients and providers develop a dark or twisted sense of humour.

Policies and Benefits

If you work or go to school, learn the rules and policies about illness and absence. At some point, you may need time off, whether a day or two here and there, or a longer stretch. Most workplaces have limits on personal or sick days, and rules about short-term disability. Find out about any documentation required. If you're a student, review the rules on absences or course withdrawals for medical reasons. Be aware of any timeframes or deadlines.

Find out what the laws in your area say about your health and employment. What information, if any, are you required to disclose to your employer about your medical condition? Can you be fired for ill health? Learn about protections available to you.

If you have an individual or group extended health insurance plan, find out what it covers. You may already have easy access to resources that could help during your treatment. Keep the plan information somewhere you can find it, so you can quickly look up details such as coverage and restrictions if the need arises.

Safety Plan

Mental illness has its ups and downs, and treatment may amplify these in the short term. Most of the downs are manageable and can wait until your next appointment. But, if your condition worsens, especially if you're contemplating any form of self-harm, it's important to address it as soon as possible. That's where your safety plan comes in.

Briefly, your safety plan outlines how to identify and resolve a crisis if it arises. Your safety plan tells you what to do so you don't need to figure it out during a crisis. Usually, you'll share your safety plan with those around you, so they, too, know what to look for and how to help.

Safety plans are customized to your unique needs. Your doctor or other mental health providers can assist you putting together your safety plan. There are examples online.[1] They typically include

- early warning signs that you may be heading into a crisis;
- coping strategies you can use to deescalate your situation early;
- ways to remove the temptation or create obstacles to prevent impulsively hurting yourself;
- people you can approach to take your mind off things or for support; and
- professionals who can help.

Crisis Resources

Finally, make sure your safety plan identifies the mental health crisis resources for your area. When you're emotional and in crisis, it is hard to think clearly enough to find the information.

If you're scared for your safety, such as feeling acutely suicidal, you need help immediately. Call your local emergency number (e.g., 911, 112, 999).

If you're with someone and you both feel you're safe enough to travel to a hospital emergency room, that's another option. Some cities centralize all emergency psychiatry services at one location. If possible, that's where you want to go. But, any hospital ER will usually do.

Finally, most regions have a mental health crisis telephone line. That doesn't replace emergency services but is one step less acute. You call and explain your situation and what you're worried about. The people who work the crisis line will help direct you to the services you need.

Hopefully, you won't need to use any of these resources, but it's better to be prepared. Make a list, as part of your safety plan or separately, and give it to friends and family just in case.

Summary

- Be sure you can take and organize notes about your appointments, gather your medical records, and look up information on the internet.
- Treatment for mental illness takes time and may involve several false starts. You'll have to persevere when people say no. You'll need to be assertive and advocate for yourself more than you're used to.
- Create a safety plan and find out about mental health crisis and emergency services in your area. You may never need them, but better safe than sorry.

7

Family and Friends

Your mental illness affects your family, friends, co-workers, and others. You may have reached out to them for support. Some people may have offered you assistance or advice out of concern for your well-being. This may or may not have been a good thing.

You may have people in your life who can help in different ways. Some may know exactly what you need and can be there to provide it. Others may not know how to help. Still others may think they're helping but are really making things worse. In theory, you can decide who joins your mental health journey and how. Realistically, some people have a hard time hearing no. It can be equally hard to ask for help.

This chapter has a few tips on how others can help you, or at least reduce the stress they're causing you.

Education

Learning about your illness is one of the best ways that people can help you. Most people don't know a lot about mental illness, and what they know may not be accurate or relevant. Learning can be something you do with them or that they do on their own.

As far as what to learn, the more conservative, mainstream, or generally accepted, the better. Those with a good foundation in the basics will be most helpful. You may have friends and family who want to share a silver bullet, a quick and easy fix. But, to be blunt, you don't need people with one-track minds nagging you to try some fantastic diet they saw on the internet. Instead, what does help are supporters who learn about your illness and the treatment options professionals suggest. You want people around to talk with who will hear what you're saying. Be aware, too, that different people learn at different rates, and mental health has a steep learning curve.

Many people may struggle to understand what's going on in your head. This is particularly true if they haven't experienced significant mental illness themselves. They're never going to know exactly what's going on, but some insight goes a long way in appreciating why you react the way you do to certain things. Being confronted with "what on earth were you thinking?" is rarely helpful to anyone. However, there is a large body of mental health writing that can help. While everyone's experience is different, many excellent books share first-person accounts of mental illness.[1]

Support

Friends and family can do many practical things to support you during your struggle with mental illness.

Very simply, they can just be there for you. They can sit with you quietly, listen when you want to talk, or give you space when you need it.

They can offer to help with daily tasks, such as doing errands, cleaning, or making dinner. Eating healthy and staying hydrated are both important. Going for walks or engaging in other forms of exercise or activities are easier to do with a partner. Encouraging connections can help, but supporters need to be mindful of the difference between offering or encouraging and pushing or nagging. Helping needs a gentle touch.

This equally applies to talking with you about your illness. It's stressful if they back you into a corner and force you to talk right then and there. It's better if they let you know they're available when you're ready. Noticing you're having a bad day and asking if you want to talk about it can be helpful. It's even better if they appreciate that "no" or "maybe later" are perfectly acceptable answers.

Keeping in mind that people just want to help, here are some useful responses when friends or family offer advice or assistance you don't need or want:

- "I greatly appreciate your help. But what I need most right now is help with…"
- "Right now, I'm just not up for discussing this. Why don't you ask again in a few days if I'd feel ready to talk then?"
- "I'm trying to simplify and not do too many things at once."
- "My doctor and I have discussed options and are working closely on treatment, but it will take some time."

Have a code word that you share with friends and family. Use it when you're out in public with them and feeling unsafe, in crisis, or extremely stressed. It's a subtle way to alert them that you are distressed without informing other people about your personal business. Discuss ahead of time how your supports should react when they hear your code word. For instance, should they take you home?

The worst thing people can do is overreact to your every word and emotion. These are not signs that things are getting worse and that your illness must be dealt with right now. Some people seem unable to resist continually offering advice though this is also unhelpful. When listening, it's usually best if people try only to listen, and not to fix what's wrong. If you do want advice or help problem solving, be very clear when is a good time for this and when is not.

Appointments

Your friends and family can also help more directly with your mental health treatment.

You may struggle during medical appointments. You may forget things you wanted to share, or have trouble answering questions or even finding the right words. You may confuse or not even hear the information, advice, or instructions given to you.

Having someone there with you can help, even if it's only to take notes. Talk with your support person about your goals for each appointment beforehand so they can remind you to bring up specific points. As an outsider, they may feel more comfortable asking clarifying questions that can help you, too. Tell them if there are certain things you want them to say or not to say.

One potential trouble spot is the transition from the pediatric to the adult healthcare system. In the former, parental involvement is encouraged and crucial. Suddenly, when you turn 18, or even before, having your parents involved is often discouraged. You've gone from having a limited say in decisions about different treatments to now being expected to make those decisions on your own. You're expected to take much more initiative and responsibility for your care. Yet, there's very little education or support to help you bridge that gap.

Afterwards, they can help you debrief and prepare for the next appointment. Reviewing material with someone else helps you better understand and remember it. They can help you update your notebook. Later in the book, we'll show you various organizational tools to keep your treatment on track. Friends and family can help with those too. They can also assist with any reading or research you need to do.

Sometimes a treatment provider might ask for someone close to you to become involved. They can provide collateral information, sharing their perspective on how you're doing. If you're comfortable with this, it can be very useful, as it is natural for people around you to notice things you don't see yourself. Sometimes family meetings can help with treatment decisions or let supporters learn how best they can help. Discuss with your provider beforehand what information they can share, and what is off limits. Family therapy (e.g., marriage counselling) can reduce conflicts affecting your mental health.

> *Summary*
>
> - Friends and family members can help in many ways, though they can also unintentionally make matters worse. Find ways to ask for help and ways to say no.
> - It's difficult to appreciate what someone else experiencing mental illness feels like, so being open to learning and available to listen are more helpful than trying to solve problems.
> - Bringing someone else to your medical appointments can be useful, but clarify their role beforehand.

8

Working With Your Family Doctor

You're all set to play a more active role in your mental health care. You're ready to learn, become more engaged in decision making, and make sure you don't get lost in the shuffle. But you can't do it alone. Your family doctor will be a critical ally on your journey.

They may be the only one helping you right now. Or, you could also be seeing a mental health specialist. If so, your family doctor's involvement shouldn't stop just because someone else is involved.

In this chapter, you'll see how working with your family doctor will improve your mental health treatment. You'll also learn how to make this relationship productive and beneficial. Keep in mind some basics:

- *Your family doctor may be the best mental health expert you have.* Psychiatrists may have greater expertise, but family doctors do most of the heavy lifting. They most likely know your whole story and understand your needs better than anyone else in the system.

- *A little knowledge is a dangerous thing.* You'll learn a good deal about mental health and its treatment in this book, but it only scratches the surface. It's no substitute for the training and experience of a good family doctor. Be open-minded. You may not have the answers.

Let's start by examining the family doctor's role in mental health care. You'll then see how their jobs have changed, leaving them struggling to manage your care the way they once did. Finally, we'll show what you can do to fill some of the gaps in care that have developed.

We're acutely aware that not everyone has a regular family doctor. Or, perhaps you have one who has less than stellar knowledge of mental health. We'll have some advice for you as well.

Roles and Responsibilities

Family doctors are the front lines of the healthcare system. They diagnose and treat problems across all areas of medicine, including mental health.

If you have an excellent family doctor, you know the difference they can make. They catch what others might miss and direct you to the most suitable treatment or resource. They go the extra mile if the situation demands it. They connect with you as a real person, somehow keeping your story separate from the hundreds or thousands of other patients they see.

Let's explore some of their roles and responsibilities in the healthcare system.

Broad Perspective

Family doctors provide a broad perspective on your health that specialists cannot. All doctors start their training by learning all areas of medicine. The surgeon with no bedside manner once worked in a psychiatry unit talking to people about their feelings. The crooked sewing job on your incision came from a student doctor who became a psychiatrist. However, family doctors are the only ones who continue to see cases covering all areas of medicine throughout their careers. They treat most routine cases and only refer some to specialists.

Mental Health Knowledge

That includes routine mental health cases. We told you earlier that mental health is involved in around 20% of all visits to family doctors. While there are many different mental illnesses, some are more common than others. Straightforward forms of anxiety and depression are seen frequently. Family doctors are far more likely to treat those and refer uncommon, severe, or exceptional cases to psychiatrists.

Family doctors are likely to be familiar with the symptoms and the typical or expected course of common mental illnesses. They're comfortable with medications such as standard antidepressants. However, some family doctors are more familiar with, capable of, and skilled at dealing with mental health problems.

Advocate

Family doctors play two crucial but complementary roles in the healthcare system: advocate and gatekeeper. As advocates, they work on your behalf to get the care you need. This includes basics such as sending you to a specialist, ordering lab tests, and prescribing medications.

Great advocates go beyond the basics. They know all the resources in your area. They might twist someone's arm to get you into a program, write letters to apply for benefit programs, or ask an insurance company to keep you on disability. They'll find shortcuts through the healthcare bureaucracy if you need them.

Gatekeeper

At the same time, family doctors keep you from getting care you don't need. In most systems, you need a referral from a family doctor to see a specialist. That way, specialists aren't flooded with minor, uncomplicated ailments, but can see the patients who most need them. Many programs with limited capacity need a doctor's referral for the same reason. Family doctors do not order unnecessary blood tests or an expensive MRI scan when a simple X-ray will do. Requiring a doctor to sign off helps keep these growing expenses slightly contained.[1]

Prioritization

Family doctors judge how acute your situation is. This affects both the care offered and how quickly you'll receive it.

They watch for signs of illnesses that need urgent treatment. If not treated, they could lead to serious injury or death. Most people know that sudden, crushing chest pain signals the immediate need for help. Family doctors recognize more subtle but still dangerous warning signs. For less acute things, they may just watch or try a few interventions, knowing that if they don't work, you're not going to be worse off for the effort.

They also prioritize referrals to specialists. How they rate the severity of your condition can make a big difference when you'll be seen. We'll talk much more about this in the next chapter.

Coordinating Care

Family doctors connect you with other parts of the healthcare system, such as specialists and labs. They make sure your care plan stays on track. They keep an eye on the big picture. If something goes awry, they'll notice and intervene. Or, that's the theory.

If this sounds a lot like patient navigation, which we discussed in chapter 5, you're right. This is one of the many things family doctors used to do but increasingly can't manage. We'll explain why next. Many of them still try to coordinate everything, but it's rarely possible. The reality is that you can no longer count on family doctors to completely guide and coordinate all aspects of your health care.

Challenges

Being a family doctor is not an easy job, and it's getting harder. There are two main reasons. Family doctors have increasing demands on their time. They also have more and more health information to keep track of. They're perpetually running behind and usually working ridiculous hours. They face alarming quantities of stress. It's no surprise that family doctors have high rates of mental illness themselves, including addiction and suicide.[2]

Something has to give. Inevitably, this will leave gaps in your care. Could you fill those gaps? (Hint: yes.) You need to understand what is being dropped. You also need to contribute in a way that doesn't make your family doctor's job more difficult. Both require a better understanding of their challenges.

Time

Increasing demands on family doctors' time results in shorter appointments and less time for other patient-related activities, such as writing a detailed referral letter or calling a colleague for advice. Your family doctor's ability to advocate for you is usually one of the major casualties. Their ability to effectively coordinate your care is another.

Information Overload

The other main challenge family doctors have is severe information overload. Doctors excel at remembering and organizing copious amounts of information. Otherwise, they'd have flunked medical school. Even so, they have limits. What's changed? Peoples' ability to process and organize information has evolved slowly over thousands of years. But, the volume of information has exploded over the last few years, thanks to computerization and the internet. It has overwhelmed everyone's ability to evolve and adapt.

Information overload is a problem for family doctors not only because of the things they don't know. It also actually changes the way they think. When there's too much information to hold in your brain at once, you naturally look for ways to simplify it. Your brain copes by focusing on the small problem in front of you. What suffers is broader, big picture thinking.

This doesn't mean your family doctor is looking at one symptom in isolation from your overall health and care plan. It does imply that broader thinking now requires a deliberate, conscious effort. This takes more time, and they are more prone to make mistakes.

Time pressures and information overload come from many places:

- *Older and sicker patients.* Demographics and medical advances have resulted in more seniors than ever before. In general, care needs rise with age, often due to chronic diseases, e.g., hypertension or diabetes. These place a growing burden on family doctors. Worse, more people now develop these illnesses at a younger age than ever before.

- *Complexity of treatment.* Medicine has not become simpler over time. New tests and medications result in better treatment for patients. Unfortunately, doctors need time to stay abreast of new information. Keeping up to date in all areas of medicine is impossible.

- *Paperwork and administration.* The amount of paperwork required of doctors has continued to grow. It's needed to order a test or comply with regulations. It's needed by specialists, employers, governments, and insurance companies. Family doctors spend several unpaid hours per day on paperwork after they finish seeing patients. Clinic practices are also changing from solo doctor to team-based care, adding to the administrative burden.

- *Electronic medical records.* Moving from paper to electronic charts has its benefits, but saving time is not one of them. You may not like your family doctor spending your whole appointment with their nose in a laptop, but they hate it even more. These programs are poorly organized and epitomize unfriendly design. They turn quick and easy tasks such as writing prescriptions into an endless stream of mouse clicks.

How Their Challenges Affect You

Not enough time in the day and too much stuff to keep track of. Who doesn't have those problems?

Don't think for a second that family doctors aren't frustrated about shortened appointments or their inability to think through your case at a deeper level. They went into medicine to help people. They'd love to do more if only they could.

So, what is being sacrificed?

- *Patient education.* What does a diagnosis mean? How will it affect you? What else could you do to help get better?
- *Managing expectations.* How long will a medication take to work?
- *Verifying comprehension.* Do you understand the question you've been asked, or the directions you've been given?
- *Thoroughness.* Are they properly reviewing your symptoms or over-simplifying questions to save time?
- *Alternatives.* Are the prescribed treatments the only options or even the ones most likely to be helpful?
- *Big picture.* Is a focus on the details causing them to miss broader fundamentals?
- *Discernment.* What are the meaningful differences between alternatives, e.g., antidepressants?
- *Up-to-date knowledge.* Is advice based on current information?
- *Optimization.* Is your care plan regularly reviewed, e.g., are medications always added, but seldom stopped?

Here are some examples of how these challenges can potentially affect your healthcare. We'll revisit a few of these in a later chapter and show how things can improve when you take a more active role in your care.

- Your doctor tries you on an antidepressant and books a follow-up in three weeks. At that visit, you complain of nausea and brain fog. They stop the antidepressant due to side effects. Because it's such a short appointment, you do not discuss that you only filled the prescription three days ago due to your anxiety. You miss out on a medication that could have worked very well once your system got used to it.
- Along with your low mood, you mention being always tired and having memory problems. They prescribe you an antidepressant and, two months later, a different one. Neither help. What they didn't do is check your iron level. They did not identify a common and easily fixed explanation for your symptoms.
- Your doctor has you try three antidepressants then gives up. Unfortunately, they were the three least likely to have helped your symptoms.
- Your family doctor recommends a counselling program, which you pay for out of pocket. Unfortunately, the type of treatment offered isn't designed to treat your form of illness.

- Your family doctor refers you to a local mental health clinic. They hold a quick intake appointment and put you in an eight-week mindfulness course. While interesting, it doesn't address your symptoms. Your family doctor meanwhile assumes the clinic took care of your mental health and doesn't pursue any other treatments.
- Your doctor refers you to a psychiatrist with a 12- to 18- month-long waiting list. When asked what to do in the meantime, they shrug and say, "I've already referred you to someone."

How You Can Help Them Help You

Your family doctor is incredibly short on time and has to keep track of information for well over 1,000 patients. You, on the other hand, may have too much time on your hands.

This sounds like a golden opportunity. If you can learn about parts of your illness and treatment, and track aspects of your care, it will free up your doctor's time. They can spend more of their time with you improving your care rather than asking or answering routine questions. Even if it takes you 25 times as long as it would take them, you've got the time and they don't. You'll still end up further ahead.

Can you learn enough from a modestly sized book like this to be helpful, without needing 10 or more years of medical education? Absolutely.

Later chapters will discuss specific things you can do to help your family doctor provide you with the best care they can. But first, here are some general principles to keep in mind as you help your family doctor help you.

Respect Their Expertise

Always remember that your family doctor is the one with the medical education and experience. That doesn't mean they're always right. But if they give you some definitive information or direction, start by assuming they know what they're talking about. You may suspect there's more to it than what they're saying. You may also doubt if they're entirely correct or up to date in an area that you've read a lot about. If so, there are good and bad ways to deal with those situations.

Good ways include asking questions:

- "Interesting. I'd like to find out more. Where do you suggest I look?"
- "I've heard other doctors approach it differently. What are the advantages and disadvantages of your approach?"

- "I trust that what you're telling me is the most likely case. Are there any other possibilities, even if more unlikely?"
- "I saw this recent article in *The Lancet*. Would it apply to me?"
- "Do you mind if I bring in what I found for us to discuss?"

But there are also bad ways to question your doctor:

- "I read on the internet that…"
- "But Dr. Phil said…"
- "My friend tried Gwyneth Paltrow's coffee enema…"[3]

Respect Their Limitations

At all times, respect their key limitations: time and information overload. If you have many things to discuss during a short appointment, be willing to schedule one or more follow-ups. If they have things they need to go through with you, preempting part of your agenda, there's a reason for that, too. Let them know your agenda items so you can plan together how to manage time most effectively.

If you've done some research, don't drop a pile of papers on them and expect them to read them. Whatever information you've found, spend some time to make it quick and easy for them to absorb. Make it concise, summarize it, or highlight the most important parts.

Keep Your Own Notes

Your family doctor takes appointment notes from their perspective. You should take notes from your perspective. As we've said, a paper notebook keeps everything in one place. It also beats having an appointment where you and your doctor spend the whole time typing instead of speaking to each other. If you keep your permanent notes in electronic form, update them after the appointment.

If you have questions, write them down before you see your doctor. That way, you'll remember them more easily during your appointment. If you get answers to those questions, information, or directions during your appointment, write them down. If you're supposed to follow up on something six months from now, write it down. Every once in a while, flip back through your notes and see if anything that should have been done was accidentally dropped.

Some people have difficulty talking, thinking, and writing at the same time. Do you feel anxious around doctors? If so, ask a friend or family member to come to the appointment with you.

If you have several people supporting you, the odds are all of them aren't going to come to every appointment. Consider keeping your notes in a shared document using tools like Google Docs. It'll save you time and energy as compared to telling everyone individually what happened. Their different perspectives might raise new ideas or questions.

Communicate Openly and Honestly

Open and honest communication is fundamental. Your family doctor is trying to help you get better. They need to know what is going on.

Be open and honest about what you're experiencing, how bad it is, and the effect it's having on you. Tell them about all your symptoms, no matter how embarrassing (they've heard it all before). Talk about the most troublesome things first. If you have many minor concerns, give them a concise, point-form list on paper that they can quickly skim. Some may seem trivial to you but may be important or raise further questions for them.

Keep your family doctor apprised of significant changes to your symptoms. This includes long-term symptoms becoming better or worse, or new things happening that weren't there before. Changes in your symptoms may suggest a progression of your illness. That might result in adjusting your treatment or even a call to the specialist to see if they could get you in sooner.

If You Don't Have a Good Family Doctor

It would be great if everyone had an excellent family doctor. But, in countless places, many people do not have a regular family doctor at all. Using the various tools and techniques in this book will be easier with a good family doctor on your side. You can use them without one, but it will be more difficult.

No Family Doctor?

For millions of people, it's impossible to find a regular family doctor. Despite that, you should still have some access to a doctor through a walk-in clinic or comparable facility in your area.

If that's your situation, try as best as you can to go to the same clinic all the time. Consider it your medical home. You may see a different doctor each time, but you will end up with a more-or-less complete medical chart there. If you receive care from other facilities, ask them to send a copy of your records to the clinic you use.

Working with a doctor who doesn't know you and may not see you again has its challenges. You need to do more work before every appointment. You need to be more concise and know what you want out of each appointment. Be explicit about your goals. Bring everything you need for them to help you. If you come across as well-prepared, confident, and organized, and make reasonable requests, most doctors will give your request serious consideration.

Family Doctor Not Up to Date on Psychiatry?

Family doctors can't know everything, and each has interests and skills in different areas. If you get the sense yours is less than current in mental health, what you'll learn here can make a substantial difference.

Without your involvement, they may be familiar with only a few treatment options, possibly ones that shouldn't be at the top of the list. They're not trying to be unhelpful. They're probably just fuzzy on the differences between various antidepressants, changes in the DSM, etc.

Bring them some logical and evidence-based suggestions along with supporting information, e.g., a medication's prescribing information. More likely than not, they'll be willing to go along with your suggestion or, at least, look into it. What they learn from you might even help with other patients.

Family Doctor Has a Bad Attitude About Anything Mental Health?

It shouldn't happen, but it does. Everyone knows there is stigma about mental health. It exists among doctors, too. Some would rather spend their time dealing with real illnesses. Others are insecure about their lack of knowledge and try to hide it. A very few think that mental illness is a made-up problem.

Patients have reported being told by family doctors, "You're fine, there's nothing wrong with you," or "Suck it up, life is hard sometimes." One recommended, "Just go to church and pray more." Some patients feel belittled or worse. Sometimes the doctors are right, and you are fine. Normal ups and downs are part of life and don't necessarily mean you have a mental illness. But they should be able to explain that to you. If you describe how your symptoms are affecting your life and you're still dismissed, this may signify a deeper problem. Talk it over with people you respect, from a variety of backgrounds. Do they think you're overreacting?

The few doctors who are openly dismissive of mental health will be hesitant to refer you to someone for help. (Sometimes though they refer quickly, so that someone else has to deal with it.) They're less likely to order tests or help you with medications, even if you present a good case. Family doctors who stigmatize patients with mental health concerns may assume everything is all in your head. Dozens of studies have concluded that people with mental illness receive poorer medical care overall.[4] That's a serious problem.

Few people have the luxury of shopping around for a different family doctor. If you are one of the lucky few, consider it. Otherwise, make the best of a bad situation. Respect their time and come in with simple, concise requests. Be appreciative when they help you a bit, even if you'd like to strangle them. Don't waste your time telling them in excruciating detail things you know they're tuning out or getting annoyed by. Find a way to a common understanding, even if it's far less than you'd like (and deserve). And keep your eyes open for other options. Is a good walk-in clinic better than what you have now?

Summary

- Family doctors train in all areas of medicine including mental health. They deal with mental health frequently and treat many cases without outside assistance.

- Family doctors have several responsibilities within a broader system. They evaluate the urgency and therefore the priority of your case, advocate for you to access certain programs, and act as gatekeepers to keep you from using scarce resources you don't need.

- Medicine has become far more complicated, and family doctors face severe time pressures, information overload, and stress. To cope, they focus more on what's immediately in front of them but have a harder time tracking the big picture.

- If you have time, you can help them with your care. For this to work, you need to have an open and honest relationship, respect their expertise, and be conscious of the difficulties they face.

9

Describing Your Symptoms

When you say "I'm depressed," you could mean many things. Maybe you're having a bad day, but maybe you're on the verge of attempting suicide.

Talking to your doctor or another provider about your mental health is not easy. Given that most doctor's appointments are short, being able to proactively, concisely, and precisely describe your symptoms is challenging but critical. Don't assume that when you use a word that your doctor will understand it the same way you do. Don't count on them to ask further questions to clarify. As an active part of your healthcare team, it's your responsibility to clearly communicate your symptoms.

Medicine has its own complex and specialized vocabulary. Ask anyone who has ever seen "SOB" written on their chart and felt offended (in medicine, it's "shortness of breath"). You don't need to learn to speak this foreign language. But you must keep in mind that what you say may not be heard the way it was intended. People often have trouble describing their mental health symptoms clearly. It's time to fix that.

Organize Your Thoughts

You're sitting across from a doctor who has just asked, "So, what brings you in today?" This is not the ideal time to start thinking about how to put your experiences and concerns into words.

Planning ahead greatly increases the likelihood that your doctor understands what's going on and why it's a problem. Writing down what you're experiencing in your notebook is a useful approach. Journalling about your symptoms each day and later summarizing them can help clarify your mental health concerns. Try to put into words what you're feeling, what's changed over time, and how it's affected your daily routine or the lives of those around you.

Speaking of which: your family, friends, and others close to you can be invaluable when trying to describe your symptoms. Often, they can articulate how you're acting or what's changed far better than you can. Ask them for feedback. They may identify patterns that you're missing.

From all this input, briefly summarize your concerns. Write them down, even in point form. If there are several different issues, pick the ones most concerning you or affecting your daily life. That way, you'll be prepared when asked, "So, what brings you in today?"

Terminology

There are hundreds of different mental health symptoms and many different ways to describe each one. We're not going to list them all here.

The important thing is to communicate each one clearly. Ideally, your descriptions should be concise—perhaps a few sentences. A lengthy and convoluted story with an evolving plot, an inspiring character arc, and several exotic locations is not a concise way to explain a symptom. Your provider may ask you to tell the story to clarify something, but don't open with it.

After listening to you describe your symptoms, your provider might say something like "Ok, that's what we call 'anhedonia.'" Great! If not, you might ask if there's a term that describes what you're experiencing. If they give you a word or phrase, fantastic! You now have some shared language. From then on, when either of you uses the word, you'll know what the other means. Write it down.

People often Google something such as, "What does depression look like?" They find a list of symptoms with brief explanations. If one seems to fit their experience, they'll use the clinical terminology to describe their symptom. On the surface, this sounds like a good idea. After all, what's more concise than a single word?

The danger is that they may not fully appreciate what the word means after just a bit of reading. A doctor may have a different idea what that word means based on their medical knowledge. Both people use the same word but mean two different things. It's better to explain what you're experiencing in your own words and then ask, e.g., "Is that psychomotor agitation?" That can get both of you speaking the same language.

Measuring Severity

Describing your symptoms precisely is important, e.g., "low mood" versus "lack of interest" versus "suicidal." Describing the severity is equally important. A mild symptom may be barely worth mentioning, while a severe one must be addressed. You can describe severity in many ways, such as by labelling symptoms "mild," "moderate," or "severe" as we've done here.

Have you ever gone to the doctor with physical pain? They've likely asked you to rate your pain on a scale of 1 (barely there) to 10 (the worst pain you can imagine). That's a useful way to describe the intensity of mental health symptoms, too. It's also a convenient way to track them over time.

Another measure is frequency. How often does the symptom affect you? Say that you're more tearful. Does this happen once or twice a week for five minutes at a time? Or is it for three hours every morning? If you're anxious, is it all the time, in particular situations, or at certain times of the day?

Finally, you can describe the impact that your symptom is having. How much is it getting in the way of your life? What is your symptom preventing you from doing? Going to work? Being in crowds? Attending your kid's soccer games? Leaving the house at all? Or, what are you doing that you usually wouldn't? Be specific. "I might be spending a bit more money than usual," is not as clear as, "I bought a boat yesterday" (assuming that is a major, unplanned expense).

Self-Rating Scales

Rating scales are a common tool used by mental health professionals. They ask you if you are having symptoms and how severe those symptoms are. Scales may come in the form of a paper questionnaire, or they may be completed via apps or on websites.

There are two types of rating scales. Clinician-rated scales are administered by a mental health professional. The professional asks you questions and writes down your answers. Usually, some interpretation is required on their part. In contrast, self-rated scales are designed so you fill them out yourself. Examples are the PHQ-9 (depression) and GAD-7 (anxiety), the latter of which is shown in Figure 9.1.

If you see your family doctor about your mental health, they may ask you to fill out one of these scales first. They use it to guide further questions or treatment options. While scales don't by themselves provide a psychiatric diagnosis, many are based on the DSM-5 (or the previous DSM-IV) criteria for different disorders. They still need to be interpreted by someone trained

9. Describing Your Symptoms

During the last 2 weeks, how often have you been bothered by the following problems?	Not at all (0)	Several days (1)	More than half the days (2)	Nearly every day (3)
1. Feeling nervous, anxious, or on edge	☐	☐	☐	☐
2. Not being able to stop or control worrying	☐	☐	☐	☐
3. Worrying too much about different things	☐	☐	☐	☐
4. Trouble relaxing	☐	☐	☐	☐
5. Being so restless that it is hard to sit still	☐	☐	☐	☐
6. Becoming easily annoyed or irritable	☐	☐	☐	☐
7. Feeling afraid as if something awful might happen	☐	☐	☐	☐

If you checked off any problems, how difficult have these problems made it for you to do your work, take care of things at home, or get along with other people?

☐ Not difficult at all ☐ Somewhat difficult ☐ Very difficult ☐ Extremely difficult

Figure 9.1: Generalized Anxiety Disorder 7-item self-report scale (GAD-7).

in mental health. You can't diagnose yourself through a questionnaire you found on the internet!

You can be proactive. You may be experiencing a variety of symptoms that suggest a particular disorder. You may have found and completed one of these self-rating scales for that disorder. Bring it with you the next time you see your doctor or other treatment provider.

You'll find links to some of the most common, freely-available self-rating scales on our website (see *Appendix A*).

Rating scales are also an excellent way to track your symptoms over time. You can compare where you were when you started treatment and where you are after a few months. Mood tracking apps are particularly convenient for this. Rating scales help to roughly quantify your symptoms at any given time and measure the effectiveness of a treatment. This is essential when reviewing your overall treatment plan. We'll describe this in detail in a later chapter.

There are many different rating scales, often many for even a single disorder. Some are freely available, while others require a fee for use. Some are more commonly used and reliable than others. Reliability, in this case, means the results of completing the scale have been statistically correlated with someone being diagnosed with a particular disorder. That is the difference between a clinically useful mental health rating scale and a quiz in Cosmopolitan magazine or a BuzzFeed listicle.

Summary

- Describing your symptoms proactively, concisely, and unambiguously is a valuable skill. It's worth taking time to think it through ahead of your appointments.

- Think about the severity of your symptoms in terms of their intensity (e.g., using a scale of 1-10), how frequently they occur, and the impact they have on your life.

- Self-rating scales can measure particular sets of symptoms, either to screen whether you potentially have an illness, or to track your progress during treatment.

10

Working the Waiting List

Some treatment providers you can approach on your own. Others need a referral. In this chapter, we'll look at referrals from your family doctor to a psychiatrist or mental health clinic. This is the most common connection between mental health providers and usually the most problematic.

As a patient navigator, you can manage connections between care providers, so that each has what they need to do their job. You can ensure appointments are booked and reports are sent, and try to minimize delays. You can even help bring new providers onto the care team.

There can be long delays before you're seen. If you must wait, there are a few tricks to help decrease the waiting time. These do not include pretending you're a politician, NHL star, or other celebrity. Some people think they are special and try to jump the queue to receive care faster than others. We're not endorsing this or any other form of lying to get ahead.

What we really want is to ensure you're in the right place in the right line. That happens less often than you might think. Human errors or omissions occur frequently. Your involvement in the process can make a difference.

We'll first explain what really happens when your family doctor refers you. Armed with a better understanding of that process, you'll learn strategies to improve the odds of getting seen sooner.

The Consultation Process

What does it mean when your family doctor says they will send you to see a psychiatrist? You've probably got a lot of questions about who you'll see, when you'll see them, for how long, etc. When your family doctor sends you to see a psychiatrist (or any specialist), this is what typically happens:

1. Your family doctor picks a psychiatrist to send you to.
2. They send a letter to the psychiatrist.
3. You (eventually) get an appointment to see the psychiatrist.
4. You go to your appointment with the psychiatrist.
5. The psychiatrist sends a letter back to your family doctor.

This is known as being referred for a consultation. Your family doctor is asking the specialist for advice about how best to help you.

Choosing the Psychiatrist

Your family doctor will have to decide who exactly to send you to. This may be, as you'd expect, an individual psychiatrist. More on that in a moment.

Services and Clinics

You may also be referred to an outpatient psychiatric service that deals with a specific type of mental health problem. It may be part of a hospital or a larger psychiatric clinic. Generally, several psychiatrists work in such a service, and you will see whichever one they decide.[1] There may be other staff who provide extra assistance and treatment. If there is a local service for your particular problem, referring you there may make the most sense.

You may also be sent to a general mental health clinic. They will normally have a psychiatrist available, but most of the staff are mental health workers such as counsellors, nurses, and social workers. You first see one of them for an intake interview about your mental health history and current needs. Based on that, you may or may not end up seeing a psychiatrist.

The Buddy System

Who your family doctor refers you to is commonly based on (in decreasing order of preference): who they have referred to before, who else they know, who other people they know recommend, and what they might find either via Google or on the website for the local medical licensing body.

In some ways, it's not a bad system. After a family doctor has sent a few patients to a psychiatrist, they can appreciate the quality of help given to their patients. They also learn a lot by asking their patients about the psychiatrist. If a past referral has worked well, they're more likely to refer again. Other family doctors, whether colleagues in the same office or those they know from elsewhere, will similarly recommend psychiatrists who they've had good experiences with. Family doctors learn over time which psychiatrists are best for different patient needs.

Your Suggestions

Your doctor may have ideas about who to send you to, but nothing is stopping you from bringing your own suggestions to them. You might find someone who can see you sooner or is a better fit. Where do you look?

You might think that the internet is a starting point. After all, every professional now has a website—except for most doctors. With few doctors and a huge demand for treatment, most don't need marketing to find patients. Some do have websites, but it's an exception.

While the doctor may be silent online, it doesn't mean their patients are. As with restaurants, teachers, or hotels, there are several online rating sites for doctors.[2] As with any anonymous review website, read user reviews with a healthy bit of skepticism. A few very good or very bad reviews probably don't mean a lot. But if enough people have commented, a pattern may emerge. Remember that your needs aren't the same as everyone else's. What other people complain about may be exactly what you're looking for.

The other way of finding a psychiatrist is by word of mouth. Fewer people will mention their fantastic psychiatrist than will talk about the beach resort where they spent their last holiday. Still, though it's one person's experience, it's better than an anonymous internet comment.

You may find a psychiatrist who looks like a good fit that your family doctor doesn't know. Don't hesitate to suggest them. Most family doctors are always looking to expand their network of reliable specialists.

Bottom line: don't hesitate to talk to your family doctor about who they're referring you to. Ask them why they made that choice and be willing to provide feedback based on things you've learned.

The Referral Letter

Your family doctor usually sends the psychiatrist a letter or fills out a form asking them to see you for a consultation. Besides your name, phone number, insurance coverage, etc., the request will ideally also include several pertinent pieces of information such as

- the problem your family doctor would like help with;
- the situation leading up to the referral, including the impact the problem is having on your life;
- specific questions or concerns they want the psychiatrist to address;
- past mental health problems, treatments, and how well they worked;
- a summary of any physical health problems;
- your current medications and doses, as well as any allergies;

- a bit about your background such as family or employment situation;
- previous reports or tests that the family doctor feels are relevant; and
- family mental and physical health history.

In spite of that, some referrals sent by family doctors literally say nothing more than, for example, "PTSD" or "ADHD." While a one-word referral (or the equally informative "Please see for PTSD") may not necessarily hurt you, it definitely won't identify you as someone who needs to be seen quickly.

Ask your family doctor for a copy of your referral letter. If it has errors, is missing or muddles your symptoms, or seems a bit skimpy, talk to them about your concern. They may ask you to give them a concise summary to pass on to the psychiatrist, or they may not change it at all. However, it won't hurt to ask.

Communication Breakdown

To be seen by a psychiatrist, their office must receive your family doctor's referral letter. You'd think this was a no-brainer. You'd be wrong.

Referrals are most often sent via error-prone 1970's-era technology (fax machines). Senders are never entirely sure what the other side has received.

The psychiatrist who received your referral might not be able to accept it. This can happen for all kinds of reasons: their practice is too full, they don't treat patients with your condition, etc. In that case (if your family doctor receives the rejection fax), it's back to square one. Another psychiatrist will be picked, and the process begins again.

Ask your family doctor how long it will take before the referral is sent. Add a healthy buffer, then check with your family doctor's administrative staff if it was sent and if they've gotten anything back. If not, call the psychiatrist's office and ask if the referral was received. Ask if they can tell you how and when you'll find out about an appointment.

Here are a few of the many things we've seen go wrong:
- family doctor starts working on a referral, puts it in a pile of paperwork to finish later, forgets it, and it never gets sent;
- family doctor puts a referral together, gives it to office staff, but it gets lost or horribly delayed in their pile of work;
- referral sits in the psychiatrist's office inbox for weeks;

- the referral is faxed, but something happens with one of the fax machines; the family doctor thinks it was sent, but the psychiatrist never gets it;
- handwritten referral is completely illegible or misinterpreted as something less serious than it is; and
- fax is sent to the wrong specialist (hint: don't refer someone to a psychiatrist to help fix their knee ligament damage).

The worst case, which is frighteningly common, looks like this:

1. Family doctor faxes your referral to the psychiatrist.
2. Psychiatrist never gets the referral (or rejects it, but the family doctor doesn't get the rejection fax).
3. Family doctor assumes you are on a waiting list and will be contacted.
4. Many months pass.
5. Family doctor's office eventually calls psychiatrist's office to ask about the status of your referral.
6. Psychiatrist's office says, "What referral?"

Don't let this happen to you!

Priorities

A concise but descriptive referral letter can make a big difference. Many psychiatrists prioritize or triage their referrals. They see the sickest people first, often before less acute cases who may have to wait longer. This is similar to what happens in the emergency room.

A good referral letter won't guarantee you get seen faster. But if your case is more serious, there's a good chance it will. If your referral just says, for example, "depression," you can bet it's getting the lowest priority. Even if they don't routinely prioritize, certain cases may occasionally still be seen before others. There are other advantages to good referral letters, which you'll see later.

Be honest about your symptoms and the effect they're having on your life. Don't minimize or exaggerate. Give your family doctor the information they need to send an accurate referral and help you. If you have old records, make sure your family doctor has them, too, so they can be passed along.

While waiting to see the psychiatrist, tell your family doctor if your symptoms change or worsen. They may send an update letter or call the psychiatrist, explain the situation has gotten worse, and ask if there's any way to bump up your appointment.

Appointment Booking

If your family doctor wrote a good referral letter, the psychiatrist received it, and you met the criteria for their practice, you're most of the way there. Ask your family doctor (or their front office staff) what happens next. Will an appointment (that may be 12 months out) be booked for you shortly? Or, will you be placed on a waiting list? Will you be given an appointment time and told to show up then, or will someone call to find a time that fits your schedule? If you will be given a specific time, who will contact you?

If you can usually be available on short notice, contact the psychiatrist's office and see if they have a cancellation list. Doctors get last-minute cancellations all the time and are always eager to fill them. This one tip can sometimes reduce your wait from a year to a month!

Make sure the psychiatrist's office knows the best way to contact you. They may only have your home phone number. So, give them your cell number if that makes sense. This is especially true if you're on their cancellation list. If you change numbers, tell both them and your family doctor.

If the psychiatrist's office publishes an email address, ask them if they prefer routine questions by email or by telephone. If you're on a waiting list, ask if it's okay to check once in a while where you are on the list. Don't overdo it. The last person you want to upset is the one booking your appointment.

You may have additional information that wasn't in your family doctor's referral letter. If you think it might be helpful to the psychiatrist, ask if it would be okay to send it to them. A one- or two-page summary of your mental health history, symptoms, medications, and past treatment providers may help. A 20-page letter detailing your current suffering will not.

> *Summary*
> - If you've been referred to a specialist, get a copy of your family doctor's referral letter. You may want to provide them with a concise summary of the crucial points to help them write it or to pass along as a supplement.
> - Try to find out about who you've been referred to. You may want to keep your eyes open for others who can see you sooner or who might be a better fit.
> - Follow up to ensure that the referral actually was received and approved by the specialist, and how and when they'll book an appointment for you.
> - If you want to be seen sooner and can be available on short notice, ask if the specialist has a cancellation list. Make sure they know the best way to reach you, especially at the last minute.

11

Mental Health Interviews

Your first visit to a psychiatrist, therapist, or mental health clinic often involves a detailed interview. A passive patient might go and assume the interviewer will cover everything. A patient who is ready to advocate for themselves and play an active role in their health care doesn't assume. You know that time pressures and information overload lead to things being missed. Preparing for the interview ensures you make the most of this opportunity.

These comprehensive interviews play a critical role. They can determine the assistance the treatment provider or clinic will offer you. They can lead to recommendations to your family doctor that may guide your ongoing treatment. Ideally, you want the suggestions to be helpful. The consultation reports that stem from these interviews also tend to follow you around. If you are referred to someone else, they'll likely get a hold of your previous reports. It helps when they're accurate.

A mental health interview is very different than speaking with most other medical specialists, such as neurologists or surgeons. In your first session, other specialists normally have a brief discussion with you about your symptoms and history. They then perform a physical exam of some sort, order a bunch of lab tests or scans and send you on your way.

Their discussion with you is important, but not very taxing. It's not something you'd likely need to prepare for. As for the rest, well, it's not like you can study for a blood test! In mental health, the discussion itself and your answers to questions play a much larger role than in other areas of medicine. You may have spent a considerable amount of time waiting to be seen. Don't let that time be wasted.

In this chapter, we'll describe what you can expect from a mental health interview, including the types of questions you will likely be asked. Jot down some notes ahead of time if you have a poor memory or anxiety. You may also want to ask family members about particular topics. Be proactive. Taking this extra initiative can result in significant benefits.

If you have an extensive mental health history (seen by many professionals, tried many medications) or a long list of physical illnesses, write it all down. A point-form list, no more than a page or two, will be helpful for the interviewer, too. Make them a copy and bring it with you.

What to Expect

As often happens when you first visit a clinic, you may be asked to complete some paperwork. They may just want your contact information or ask questions about your physical and mental health history. They may ask you to complete some of the self-rating scales we discussed earlier.

You then meet with the psychiatrist, psychologist, social worker, nurse, or other provider conducting your interview. Don't be surprised if they get right down to business. Some will spend a few minutes to help you feel comfortable and explain what will happen during your appointment. Others introduce themselves (hopefully) and start asking questions.

Mental health interviews consist of a lot of questions, often deeply personal. Usually, the interviewer steers the conversation to keep your answers short. That way they have time for all their other questions. Being on the receiving end of this questioning can be intense, especially if you're not expecting it. Some people describe it as facing a verbal machine gun.

If you don't think well on your feet, this may feel overwhelming. As well, many people are understandably anxious during these appointments. Let the interviewer know about your anxiety or any other difficulty you're having. They may be able to adjust their interviewing style to help you. They might also bring you back for a second appointment to complete the initial interview; but, for many reasons, this isn't often possible.

These interviews pack a lot into a short time. You may have other information to share, to provide a fuller answer or add what you feel is the necessary background. Sometimes you may feel like you're getting cut off, as the interviewer tries to manage the time. Help them by pointing out your biggest concerns, saying, for example, "This has been a huge problem," and, "Let's return to it later" if they pressure you to move on. Feeling frustrated is common. After all, you're faced with a barrage of highly personal questions, posed by a person you just met. Try not to get your back up.

Keep in mind that the interview is for your benefit, and not for the person interviewing you. Doing some preparation beforehand can be a big help. The diagnosis and treatment advice the interviewer will eventually give are only as good as your answers. The rest of this chapter will show you the types of questions likely to be asked.

Why the big rush? It's all about time. Many clinics only set aside a certain amount of time for each new patient. Often this is how long it would take to interview an ideal patient. Ideal means someone with a straightforward history and problem who can communicate with ease.

Practical considerations such as the number of staff in the clinic affect how much time is available. Many clinics have goals for the number of patients they're supposed to see. Another factor is the amount of time they're willing to lose if someone doesn't show up for their appointment. This, unfortunately, happens more often than you'd think. When it comes to psychiatrists, there's another reason—billing. In many places, they're paid a fixed amount, no matter how much or how little time they spend on a consultation. As a result, most psychiatric consultations tend to be around 45–50 minutes in length.

That's not a lot of time to share your whole story with a person you've just met, who is asking questions you may never have thought about before. If you think this sounds more like a job interview or university exam than a medical appointment, you're not entirely wrong. Did we mention that preparation can help?

Typical Questions

Mental health interviews tend to follow a regular pattern, though usually adapted to your situation. They might focus more on some areas and omit or skim through others. There is no completely standard interview, and interviewers have their own quirks. Still, conducting a comprehensive but efficient interview is part of mental health training.

You may not be asked some important and highly relevant questions. Often, the interviewer already has the answers from other sources such as an excellent referral letter or material your family doctor sent along with it. Other sources include previous consultations, labs, or medication lists pulled from an electronic medical record. The interviewer may quickly verify the information with you, but given the time pressure, usually not.

Basics

The interviewer's job is to get a picture of who you are. This starts with information such as your age and gender (which may encompass biological gender, gender identity, gender expression, sexual orientation, and much more). They may also ask things such as:

- Are you currently single, married, living common-law, or divorced? Do you have a regular romantic partner? Has anything changed recently?
- Do you have children?
- Where do you live, and who else lives there with you?
- What do you (or did you) do for work, school, or other important areas of your life?
- What is your current source of income?

Current Illness

You've sought help and are now in this interview for a reason. So, the interviewer will want to know more about your symptoms and may ask:

- How would you describe your current difficulties?
- How long have you been experiencing these difficulties?
- Are they getting worse? How have they progressed over time?
- How is your illness impacting your life?
- Were there any events that you think triggered the problems?
- What would being better look like?

If someone is going to help you, they need to know what exactly they're helping you with! They may also ask what you hope to get out of this interview, to ensure that your expectations line up with theirs.

Mental Health History

The interviewer will ask about your past mental health history. Your past experiences are invaluable in assessing your current situation. Knowing what treatments have or haven't worked in the past also helps narrow down further treatment options. Your formal mental health history covers any periods of time when you saw a mental health professional. For each, consider the following:

- What caused you to seek help?
- Who did you see?
- How long/often did you see them?
- What diagnosis (or diagnoses) were you given, if any?

- What treatments were tried (e.g., psychotherapy, medications)?
- What helped? What didn't help?
- If you tried medications, why were they stopped?

Your history includes the times you were admitted to hospital for mental health reasons. It includes visits to the ER for mental health symptoms, voluntarily or not. It also includes any previous suicide attempts, self-harm (e.g., hair pulling, cutting), or harming anyone else (e.g., legal history). The interviewer may request your records from previous treatment providers to fill in gaps. Some records may have been sent with the referral.

Your mental health history also encompasses mental health struggles when you weren't seen by a professional. Many people battle for months, years, or decades before seeking help. Providers want to know what problems you had and how they affected you. They also want to know how you coped, including unhealthy coping such as self-harm or self-medicating with alcohol or drugs.

Physical Health

Your mental health is intricately tied to your physical health. Your mental health providers need to understand your physical health history and current issues. Even if you are seeing a counsellor or psychologist, who won't have had the medical training of a doctor or nurse, they need to know about this.

Your physical health impacts your mental health in so many ways. Some physical illnesses directly cause mental health symptoms. Many medications for physical illnesses do the same thing. Struggling psychologically with a physical illness can also lead to mental health problems. Your physical health may also affect what mental health treatments are safe to use. Even things that might sound innocuous to you may not be. Let your provider know everything and let them sort out what is relevant. Include both current and past physical health problems.

Medications and More

The interviewer will ask about the medications you're currently on. That includes mental health medications but also others. So many medications interact with one another that it pays to be safe. They also want to look out for medications that can trigger mental health symptoms. You should include over-the-counter, and herbal or natural products too. Many of these can also interact with prescribed medications or can affect mental health. Report any allergies or sensitivities, especially to medications.

You will also likely be asked about substance use, both perfectly legal and illegal, and how much you use. Such substances include
- caffeine (e.g., coffee, tea, cola, energy drinks, some exercise supplements), which often increases anxiety;
- nicotine (smoking, chewing, vaping);
- alcohol;
- cannabis (including strain and/or CBD:THC ratio); and
- other street drugs.

We'll talk about how different substances can affect mental health later in the book.

Family History

There is a strong genetic component to some mental illnesses. Having a relative with a mental illness may increase your risk of developing that illness or a related illness. It can help to know about past or current mental illness in biological family members, including
- anxiety or depression;
- schizophrenia;
- bipolar disorders;
- addictions issues;
- personality disorders;
- suicides (or attempts);
- hospitalizations (a marker of the severity of their illness); and
- treatments (medications, therapy, etc.) they used and how well they helped because something that helped a relative has a greater chance of helping you.

Not all families are equally open about mental illness. It's common that even when there is a history of mental illness, nobody in the family talks about it or seeks treatment for it. Often, you're pretty sure that a family member has an undiagnosed mental illness. If your family doesn't talk about it, it's better to tell the interviewer that you suspect something rather than deny your relative has had a mental illness. If you are adopted, mention that, and whether you know details about your biological family.

Learning about your family mental and physical health history can help you now and in the future. If you haven't had the conversation, it's worth having. If your family doesn't know or says they don't want to talk about it, don't worry. They may be more open later. Attitudes can and do change, often after the death of a strong family matriarch or patriarch.

Social History

Your social history includes where you were born, where you lived, your time with your family during childhood, schooling, relationships, etc. Yes, this includes the cliché, "so tell me about your mother." This can help the interviewer to understand your overall story and even identify past events affecting you now.

Certain behaviours and ways of coping with stressors are developed very early in life and affect your behaviour. Experiencing traumatic events can also have long-term consequences. It's not uncommon to see PTSD misdiagnosed as another form of anxiety.

Typical Day

You may be asked to describe a typical day. This is another way for the interviewer to learn how your illness may be impacting you. Sometimes you may not even consciously realize how it affects you. You might think that most people think or act the same way you do. Describing your day can reveal things that asking about your symptoms won't, and so the interviewer may ask

- how much you sleep, if you wake up often, have nightmares, don't feel rested, or sleep during the day;
- how much energy you have;
- what activities you participate in or how much you stay at home;
- if you eat in a healthy and nutritious manner, and exercise;
- what stressors may be impacting your life; and
- your key relationships.

Symptom Screen

The interviewer will ask you about other symptoms that haven't come up earlier in your discussion. We discussed this in the *Describing Your Symptoms* chapter, but typical examples include

- depressive symptoms (e.g., low mood, lack of interest or motivation);
- *hypomania* or *mania* (i.e., an abnormally elevated mood lasting at least several days, often with severe irritability, grandiosity, lack of

sleep, faster speech, racing thoughts, excess energy or activity, and poor judgment; hypomania is a milder form of mania);
- psychotic symptoms (e.g., hearing voices);
- different types of anxiety (e.g., future-oriented worry, obsessive-compulsive rituals, social anxiety);
- sleep disturbances;
- eating disorders (e.g., binge, purge);
- gambling or other addictive behaviours;
- concentration, memory, attention, learning disability; and
- suicidal or homicidal thoughts, intent or plans.

Some of these may have been covered by self-report scales that you completed earlier. Time restrictions sometimes result in screening questions that are too brief. We've heard of some providers screening for hypomania or mania by asking only, "Do you ever spend too much money?" That's cutting a few too many corners. Obviously, if you have major concerns that weren't directly asked about, make sure to bring them up.

Follow-Up

At the end of the interview, make sure you know what the next steps are. Will you be meeting with the interviewer again? If so, when? Do you need to set up an appointment?

Will a report be sent back to your referring doctor? If so, how long should that take? Plan to make an appointment with the doctor who referred you shortly thereafter.

Summary

- Mental health interviews are more involved than when you see other types of medical specialists. They pack a lot into a short time. Some advance preparation, including making notes, can help you get the most out of them.
- Common topics include what problems you're currently having, any past mental health problems or treatments, your physical health, medications, supplements, substance use, any family mental health problems, a bit about how you grew up, what a typical day is like, and whether you're experiencing any of a very long list of symptoms.
- Afterwards, find out what happens next. Who will you see and when?

12

Difficult Encounters

This is one of those chapters we'd rather not write or only include as a brief paragraph. But given how many people have had negative experiences with mental health care, we can't ignore this topic.

The people who treat you are skilled professionals. Most are caring and genuinely want to help. They want to see you healthy again. Ideally, they are friendly, empathetic, respectful, reassuring, and even delightful.

Unfortunately, this isn't always the case. Some people don't have a good experience with a mental health provider. Others find the experience unhelpful. A few find it so horrific that it leaves them traumatized years after.

Sometimes this is due to unrealistic expectations. You hope you've finally found the person who can help get your life back on track. Instead, they're doing their best to get through their sixth interview of the day and not confuse your story with that of someone else. At other times, patients don't know what to expect at all. That won't be the case for you after reading the previous chapter. The person interviewing you may be cold, rude, or belligerent. In an ideal world, you could walk out the door and immediately see someone else. Unfortunately, it doesn't work that way.

Taking charge of your mental health means knowing the system, warts and all, and making the most of each opportunity. Preparing for what could be an uncomfortable (or worse) interview is part of taking charge. It can keep a bad situation from getting worse or salvage a futile interview. We hope this isn't something you need to use. Still, forewarned is forearmed.

In what follows, we'll introduce you to a motley crew of unsavoury characters you may have the misfortune to meet. These are all based on actual events that patients have shared with us. Afterwards, we'll offer some general advice for dealing with these and other situations.

The Nasty Sourpuss

Everyone knows this character. From the start, they're gruff, frustrated, or rude. You're sure they woke up on the wrong side of the bed and found that someone peed in their corn flakes. Not the welcome you'd expect from someone whose job is to help people who often feel vulnerable and scared.

They might always be a grumpy jerk, or, most likely, they're having a bad day. They may be ill or have a sick kid. They might have had an argument with their spouse or had a colleague yell at them. It's your bad luck that their crappy day coincides with the one day you see them.

It's not easy being the target of someone else's bad day. Rest assured it's most likely caused by something else. Healthcare is a stressful environment. People become jaded. Sometimes they take it out on you. All you can do is remind yourself that it's them, not you, and deal with it the best you can.

The Slow Starter

You waited months or years for this appointment, worried about it for days. You hope it will turn your life around. You're seeing the expert now. They enter, quickly glance at the consult letter, apparently for the first time. They ask, "So, what are you here for?" Your heart drops.

This may be a once-in-a-lifetime visit for you, but it's just another day in the office for them. They're constantly seeing new patients. Some specialists prefer to start with your perspective and integrate what your referring doctor had to say afterwards. Others know that, because of the long wait time, your situation has likely changed from what your family doctor told them.

Everything won't be resolved in the first ten seconds. This is a marathon, not a sprint. But, if things are still off-track after ten minutes, clearly tell them what you expected from this visit. Try to get on the same page.

The Sprinter

We talked earlier about mental health interviews being akin to machine-gun questioning. Some providers are undeniably more set than others on getting through everything in the time they have with you. They may get irritated if you don't answer fast enough or say too much.

You are discussing some intensely personal experiences. You may have never shared them before and are now telling them to a complete stranger. It's a bit presumptuous to expect you can rattle off answers as if you're reading a grocery list. And more than a little bit rude. Do your best, try to keep calm, and do not get your back up. Many times, the interview is the start of a longer process. You'll have other opportunities to tell more of your story.

The One-Track Mind

Any doctor can have their particular hang-ups, things they emphasize just a bit too much. Your family doctor might focus on smoking, exercise, and diet. It's not that these aren't important, but continually harping on them wears thin after a while. If they really ignore everything else and only focus on their hot buttons, it affects the quality of your care.

Mental health professionals aren't immune to this. Some might obsess over caffeine intake. Yes, cutting back on caffeine if you're anxious is a good start, but only part of the problem. Others insist that certain medications (e.g., benzodiazepines) should never be used and focus on that. Some will refuse to deal with anything else until alcohol or drug problems are resolved. (Incidentally, most guidelines recommend concurrent treatment of addiction and other mental health problems.)

The Very Specialized Specialist

You wouldn't expect a psychiatrist to say, "Depression? I don't treat depression!" It can happen though. Many have general practices, seeing a bit of everything, e.g., anxiety, depression. Some sub-specialize and focus on one area of mental health. It does sound odd for a psychiatrist to say, "I'll treat your ADHD, but you'll have to see someone else for your depression." But in some areas, such as eating disorders, there are so few psychiatrists relative to the demand, it does happen. This is another reason why you and your family doctor should check out who you're being sent to ahead of time. Their practice may not be appropriate for your needs.

The Really Alternative Practitioner

Some people take specialization to a whole different dimension. There are a few psychiatrists, fully trained and licensed, who have a less-than-mainstream focus in their practice. This isn't about only treating ADHD or eating disorders. They treat people exclusively using the incredible wisdom found in a particular book. Eckhart Tolle and Deepak Chopra tend to be popular, as are the Bible or other religious texts. Or perhaps they see everything through a very narrow-focus lens. A psychiatrist who attributes all mental health problems to trauma related to abortion is an example.

These people may be trained, qualified, and licensed as psychiatrists, but they're not in any way practicing as psychiatrists. Run.

The Not Really a Psychiatrist

We had one patient who saw the same psychiatrist on three occasions. Their reports gave a different diagnosis each time. Two of the three diagnoses were not actually from the DSM-5 or previous editions. The assessments also didn't appear to meet the standard of practice for psychiatrists. They missed essential elements like whether the patient was suicidal.

We did some digging and found that this doctor completed psychiatric training in another country. However, they had not yet met the national standards of practice qualifying them as a specialist in psychiatry in Canada.[1] But they had a medical license and could practice psychiatry here. They were always called "the psychiatrist." Nobody knew differently.

The Diagnostic Nerd

Some specialists are obsessed with the diagnosis. Clarifying a diagnosis is often one of the main reasons that family doctors refer to psychiatrists. Diagnosis is important, but for some psychiatrists, it's really important. Their one mission is making sure the diagnosis is exact, precise, with every specifier correctly quantified.[2] If they can diagnose a rare or obscure illness, they may need a cold shower before seeing their next patient.

Both you and your family doctor are probably interested in the psychiatrist's opinion of your diagnosis. But what you truly want to know is how to get better. Keep in mind that getting the right diagnosis is itself a valuable step toward finding the right treatment.

The Psychic

Some providers have you pegged the moment you walk into the office. At the outside, it takes five minutes of talking with you. A full interview is a pointless waste of their time.

It's sheer arrogance to think anyone could learn everything relevant about you in a single visit. Most people don't completely open up the first time they meet someone. Giving someone a superficial diagnosis after a few minutes in an unfamiliar environment is unprofessional and demeaning. The full story is often needed to appreciate the situation. Many illnesses have significant areas of overlap that take time to distinguish. A token interview does you and the doctor who referred you a disservice.

People with distressing mental health conditions often have more than one thing going on. Proper treatment takes this into account. Treating what's merely on the surface is a guarantee you'll be seeking care again in the not-too-distant future. Welcome to mental health's revolving door.

The Expert Know-It-All

Everybody experiences mental illness differently. So, what to make of the expert who thinks they know what's going on in your head based only on your diagnosis? Or, who definitively says that you aren't experiencing what you describe? They may have treated 500 patients with a bipolar illness. Then you come along with some symptoms that are slightly different. It doesn't mean you're not experiencing them. When their mental model doesn't fit a new piece of data (i.e., you), you're not necessarily wrong. They may know more than you about psychiatry, but you know more than they do about what you're actually experiencing.

Sometimes though, it turns out they are right. A symptom you thought was due to medication sensitivity may be anxiety about taking it. Worsening of your symptoms may not be related to your treatment but to a new life stressor. The best psychiatrists don't tell you they're right or you're wrong. Instead, they'll share how most people react, acknowledging that everyone is different. It's an opportunity to consider alternatives. Maybe something else is going on. If both of you can keep an open mind moving forward, you may reach a better understanding.

The God Complex

At the extreme, some people feel they are so brilliant that they don't need to take what you say into account. They'll listen to you only if it's a direct answer to one of their questions. Consider yourself lucky that you've been permitted to bask in their presence. They look down on patients as people who are beneath them, and certainly not equals. Patients are almost like objects that can be manipulated. These providers are condescending and paternalistic. They'll tell you the way things really are. Any advice you've gotten from anywhere else is wrong. It doesn't matter if it comes from other specialists or your family doctor who you have known your entire life. This attitude, sadly, can be found in nearly every profession and setting.

The Complete Jerk

And of course, some people treat everyone they see badly. The reasons—arrogance, prejudice, stigma, or whatever—it really doesn't matter. You're an imposition, a waste of their time. You're stupid. You are the cause of all your own problems. You're completely broken, and there's nothing that anybody can do to fix it. While it's bizarre to find people like that in a caring profession, unfortunately, there are some. Hopefully, you won't ever encounter one of them.

Our Advice to You

The above characters are exceptions. Most mental health workers, though stressed and frazzled, are kind and considerate. But they are human. These extreme examples are a minority. With luck, you'll never meet them.

Some of the behaviours we described, if not mean or abusive, are at the very least quirky or unusual. We think it's best that you're aware these people are out there in case you do encounter them. Being surprised and taken aback could derail the interview. Look at it this way. High expectations are rarely surpassed. Low expectations are often exceeded. Your choice.

We recognize the inherent power imbalance in these situations. You need them, or at least their expertise, a lot more than they need you. That's no excuse for bad behaviour, and no reason to put up with abuse. You can be polite, respectful, and assertive at the same time. However, there is nothing to gain by antagonizing them. Resist pushing back when emotions run high. Decide which battles to fight and when to grit your teeth and move on.

Having said all that, we offer you the following advice for any interview:

- Be on time.
- Be prepared. If there are things you've been asked to bring, show up with them. If you have other information, bring a copy to leave. Think about how to answer the questions in the previous chapter.
- Gently remind them of your goals. Get on track early.
- Remember that the interview is for your benefit, not the interviewer's. Be honest, open, and straightforward. Provide the best information you can. You're more likely to get useful advice in the end.
- You're not there to make friends. Some people want everyone to like them. Watch out if you're one of those people. If the provider is rude, insulting, or arrogant, try your very best not to get your back up.
- You're there for an opinion and advice. You should consider it seriously, but you don't have to agree with it or act on it.

Summary

- Even though most are not, some people can be real schmucks. That includes people who work in mental health.
- It's in your best interest to try to be as helpful as possible, no matter what you think of the interviewer or their behaviour. Even the vilest person may have something useful to offer.

13

Paging Dr. Google

Long before you spoke with your family doctor or anyone else about your mental health concerns, you likely looked online. Your search introduced you to a flood of scary diagnoses. Google searches on each diagnosis then revealed some pretty astounding "cures." You surely found dire predictions for what remains of your (now greatly shortened) life. Did you look up a medication someone recommended? The horror stories you found would make Stephen King or H.P. Lovecraft proud. If you didn't have anxiety problems before, a few hours of internet searching would have changed that.

In the good old days, before about 1993, doctors had all the answers. Not anymore. Patients have more information, questions, and suggestions than ever. No matter how many doctors might like to put the genie back in the bottle, it's not going to happen. If you're taking a more active role in managing your care, you'll need to do some research. The ability to locate relevant and accurate information is critical.

You can find almost anything on the internet, and that's the problem. You'll find a lot of both good and bad health information. There's also a whole lot of money to be made by selling you health-related products. There's no shortage of credible-looking information carefully designed to convince you that you have a disease. The same information will tell you, surprise, surprise, that their brand of snake oil will cure that disease.

Your doctor probably uses Google too, though not necessarily in your presence. It's a speedy way to access information, much faster than flipping through books and journals. The difference is, they know how to separate the reliable information from all the rest. It's time for you to learn to do the same. We'll first show you how to improve your searching to initially filter what you find, and then we'll touch on the limitations of clinical evidence.

Credibility

It's important to consider the source of any information, especially if you found it online. It's generally understood that medical information from the Mayo Clinic, the US Food and Drug Administration (FDA), the UK National Health Service (NHS), or Health Canada is more trustworthy than something from a random website. Separating out credible from crap is rarely that straightforward. Here a few credibility traps easy to fall into:

- *Fake journals.* Historically, academic journals have published quality information. However, there are more and more journals whose content is neither edited nor reviewed. Instead, authors pay to have their material published. Authors hope this lends a veneer of credibility that will deceive the public. These journals have names and branding similar to reputable journals. Unfortunately, if you're not an expert in the area, it's hard to know the difference. Some resources can help.[1]

- *Non-medical university sites.* Medicine faculties in universities worldwide publish some great information. But just because something comes from a university does not guarantee its credibility. Be suspicious of information published individually rather than by a medical department. Also, be wary of medical advice coming from non-medical departments of a university. Pronouncements on psychiatry posted by one person from an education faculty likely do not provide a good basis for clinical choices.

- *Fake or discredited experts.* Be wary of people who promote themselves as experts but who are not. They may no longer be affiliated with professional institutions or have been discredited. Searching for their names can corroborate their credentials. It can also reveal controversies or other reasons why they're no longer considered credible.

- *Media stories.* Health stories in the media focus on new treatments and innovations. They are an invitation to explore further. The information they provide should be considered in a broader evidence-based context, not alone. Most stories are drastic simplifications of the facts and omit vital information. They skip details that might offer a clue as to whether the story may be relevant to you. Many media stories come straight from press releases issued by the people in the stories. Modern journalists are stretched so thin that it is rare for them to spend the time to provide the context and detail you need.

- *Social Media.* There are thousands of social media groups on mental health, many of which have very knowledgeable participants. But don't act on advice you read there or base your research only on the recommendations you find in those groups. Groups tend to attract like-minded people. Even if something has massive support in a certain online community, it's highly unlikely to be representative of the range of expert opinions you'd want to rely on.

- *Sales Materials.* Finally, be wary of websites with studies or other information about a product they sell. This is particularly true of natural health products. The industry has few codes of conduct or rules about truth in advertising. At least keep pharmaceutical companies are kept on a bit of a leash by regulators like the FDA and Health Canada.

Independent Validation

In science, including medicine, in general, independent validation is critical. If only one person or company makes a claim, don't rely too heavily on that claim. Errors, omissions, bias, or even deception can undermine the claim. Validation tackles this problem by inviting other researchers to conduct studies that will either support or refute the claim. When multiple independent parties can make the same claim, you can have more confidence in its validity.

Independent validation relies on the credibility of all parties making a claim. If one is not credible, their support adds nothing to the claim. Independence can sometimes be difficult to verify. Different people or research groups may work for the same organization or receive funding from a common source. People may be former colleagues. They may be part of a fringe group whose methods and conclusions are well outside the mainstream.

> Anti-psychiatry is an excellent example of a position taken by some fringe groups. These groups are made up of many different people from different institutions and disciplines. They all make very similar claims about psychiatry. They think it is a cruel, corrupt, and unjust practice focused on state control of dissent. They believe mental illness does not exist. They want all treatments abolished.
>
> Look closer, and you see the same group of writers making the same group of claims. They generally reference one another to lend support to the claims. Critically, there is little intellectual engagement with the much larger mainstream psychiatry and mental health community. Such an echo chamber reflects a very limited, isolated, and self-reinforcing worldview. That is the opposite of independent validation.

Don't hesitate to ask your care providers their thoughts on articles you've found. Ask them to recommend articles, journals, or other resources to explain a topic. You may find newer information using these same sources that your doctor is not aware of.

Lies, Damn Lies, and Evidence

Before proceeding, we'll let you in on a secret about evidence. People tell you a treatment they want you to use has been proven successful through evidence. Doctors and other professionals may use an evidence-based approach. Science gives us objective confidence through evidence.

Evidence is important. However, hearing there is evidence for a treatment often does not mean what you think it means. We'll explain, but here's the bottom line:

If someone says there is evidence that 'X' will treat your mental illness, there is a high probability that it will be of little help to you.

Most people need to try several different treatments before they find one or more that fully treats their illness. Evidence doesn't predict what will work. Science doesn't provide the certainty many people want. Here's why:

- Evidence isn't an absolute. There are different levels of evidence, some stronger than others. This is true in all areas of medicine.

- Mental health research is tricky because mental illness is so complicated. Illnesses are made up of many possible symptoms, each of which may have a multitude of different causes. Studies can show a treatment helps those with a certain illness, even if it only affects some symptoms or causes. These may not apply to you.

- Stronger evidence results from limiting variability. To reduce variability, experiments may exclude people who have other physical or mental illnesses, people of certain ages, social backgrounds, etc. But mental health symptoms are affected by many factors, often intertwined. Limiting variability may produce stronger evidence, but the results may apply to very few people.

Thorough testing that takes into account the variability found in the real world is practically impossible. Tools to examine and measure results are also limited. Evidence in mental health, therefore, has more caveats. Evidence cannot reliably predict what will or won't work for someone. It's not like evidence in chemistry class where all you're checking is to see if adding A to B turns B purple. Evidence in mental health is no guarantee.

If you want a deeper understanding of why evidence in mental health is less clear-cut, we've posted an in-depth article on this topic on our website (see *Appendix A*). It covers different types of studies and their associated levels of evidence, the quality of evidence, and explains certain technical meanings of everyday words such as "significant." It also covers in great detail how study design is forced to hide so much of the variability underlying mental illness, even when what's being hidden is very relevant to interpreting the evidence. It explains, despite these limitations, how to best incorporate mental health evidence into your own treatment.

This will also help if you need to argue with people about treatments. Compelled to justify why you're not drinking 10 cups of tea each day made from a stinky plant that a persistent relative pulled from their garden? Go read the article. Or get them to read it. While they're drinking their tea.

Applicability

You've found some medical information that appears to be from a credible source. The best question you can then ask is, "Does this apply to me?"

Hearing that something is a "fantastic treatment" is meaningless. You need to know what condition the treatment is for and who it has been shown to help. You may need to dig deep to find answers. It's human nature to believe or claim something is more widely applicable than it is. Which of these two claims would a salesperson rather make? Which could possibly be true?

- This treatment will help everyone with any mental illness.

- This treatment will help improve one symptom that occurs in 3.5% of all people diagnosed with major depressive disorder but was only tested on adult males aged 25–35 with no other medical problems.

Who does this medical information apply to? How does this treatment compare to other treatments? Are these other treatments ones you might be considering? If these details aren't there, ask yourself why.

Shiny and New

Everyone gets excited by the latest breakthrough. But when it comes to your own health, do you really want shiny and new? Or, do you want something slightly older but better understood? To put it another way, do you want to be a guinea pig?

The media likes reporting on the latest technologies and innovations. They are newsworthy. Another study of a well-known medication confirming it is safe and helpful is not as appealing to media. The drawback of trying the latest thing is that there are many unknowns. A new study finding an unexpected result needs to be independently validated and analyzed. Its findings may or may not stand up to scrutiny.

A newly approved medication may promise exciting and significant benefits over existing treatments. Testing during its development likely involved only a few hundred people over a few months. With an established medication, thousands or millions of peoples' experiences reveal rare side effects and long-term impacts. Over time, concerns may arise about using it in some people, e.g., it can worsen another health condition. New insights into prescribing are learned. These improve effectiveness or tolerability.

We're not suggesting you never take a new medication or participate in a new treatment program. But it almost always makes more sense to rely on established treatments first. If several standard treatments haven't worked, then start looking at newer options. Recognize that newer options carry some degree of increased risk.

Companies are eager to showcase how their newest medications are better than older generation products. It's not only about the novelty of newer treatments. It's also about profits.

New medications are covered by patents that protect intellectual property for several years. The length of time varies by country. During that time, no other company can sell a version of the same medication. If you've got a blockbuster medication on your hands and you're the only one who can sell it, you're going to make a tonne of money.

After patent protections expire, other companies can sell their versions of the medication. These *generics* are often much cheaper than the original *brand name* medication. When the original monopoly ends, profits will tumble.

If the company releases a new medication for the same condition, that new medication will be protected by new patents. The monopoly clock starts all over again. It's no surprise to see new medications released just as the patents for old ones expire. Some are genuine innovations that greatly differ from the older medication. Others are only minor reformulations, but still different enough to be patented. The company's profits now depend on the ability to sell the new medication rather than the old one. They will trumpet any benefit, no matter how small, as a world-changing innovation.

Confirmation Bias

When researching an illness or treatment, be very conscious of *confirmation bias*. This is the tendency to place higher value on information that agrees with your existing beliefs and to devalue material contrary to existing beliefs. We all do this to some degree, usually unconsciously.

Say that you've heard good things about a medication, maybe read a couple of positive articles. You may be inclined to believe it has a lot of potential to help you. Based on that belief, you're more likely to notice other articles that reinforce your belief. You'll also consider those same articles to be of higher quality. In contrast, you will tend to skip articles that show negative aspects of the medication. You may feel they are weaker articles.

Confirmation bias exists in many areas of life—politics and music to name two. When it comes to your health, you want to use the most objective evidence that you can find. You want to accurately appreciate the benefits and risks. You can't avoid confirmation bias, but you can be conscious of it.

Google Scholar

Everyone knows Google's web search. A far lesser-known tool is Google Scholar (scholar.google.com).

Google Scholar doesn't search the entire web. Instead, it searches only reputable academic journals and similar publications. For reliable medical information, this is a gold mine. Finding information in a reputable journal is a good step forward. But it gets better.

Academics build on the work of other researchers. They carefully put their contribution in context, comparing and contrasting it with existing work. This is reflected in the lengthy reference lists at the end of academic papers. For each paper, Google Scholar tracks which other papers it references. It can answer questions such as, "How many other papers have referenced this one?" A paper referenced by 1,000 other papers has something important to say, good or bad. A paper that few others have referenced could just be very new. If not, it doesn't have a lot important to say, at least as far as influencing understanding within its field.

Google Scholar makes it easy to follow these chains of references. You can identify key papers and see how they are regarded by other authors. For papers published several years ago, you might find newer or updated information. It may either support or refute the information in the original paper. Used wisely, Google Scholar can ensure what you read is relevant, credible, and reflects the best current understanding.

Unfortunately, the entire paper may not be available to view or it may require a fee. Some papers can only be read by people or institutions that pay for pricey journal subscriptions. In other cases, you can pay for individual papers yourself. Without paying, you may only see the title, authors, publication details, and abstract.

Sharing What You've Learned

You've seen many ways that dialogue with your treatment providers can improve your care. This also applies when sharing information that you've found online. You may introduce them to new ideas helpful in your case and perhaps even with some of their other patients. They may gain insight into how you're thinking about your illness and the questions you have. At the same time, they may help you by providing further context based on their training, research, and experiences. They can help you apply general information to your specific situation. Often, the back-and-forth will lead in a new and promising direction.

You may be excited about what you've found. But, the odds of it being an undiscovered silver bullet are slim. Don't approach your treatment providers with the intent of dictating a new plan solely based on an internet search. Instead, think about having a discussion. How does this new information apply? Bring a copy of your research to give to them. Highlight some of the most relevant bits. Be prepared to concisely summarize it. At the same time, don't insist they talk about it right then and there. The most open-minded doctor may have other things they need to complete during your appointment. Most importantly, when they do discuss it, listen to what they say just as you expect them to listen to what you say.[2]

> ### Summary
>
> - You can find almost anything on the internet, but finding high-quality information that's relevant to your situation can be extremely difficult.
> - Obstacles you'll face include people making claims to sell you things; difficulty identifying credible sources of information that have been independently validated; and, applying the information to your unique situation.
> - Newer isn't always better, especially in medicine.
> - Google Scholar can drastically narrow your search and help you separate an oddball theory from widespread clinical practice.

14

Your Living Treatment Plan

Keeping your treatment from stalling or going astray can be a challenge. This chapter gives you a powerful tool to prevent that.

Going off in different directions at each appointment isn't good care. To avoid this, you need a current and up-to-date plan. It should reflect everyone's best understanding of your illness and treatment. We call this a *living treatment plan* because it grows and changes over time. It is a plan that is easily updated and that everyone works from.

A living treatment plan maps out your care, showing both the big picture and details. It tracks the best available treatment options and how to implement them. It ensures you use your time wisely and focus on treatments that are working. If you're waiting for a specialist, getting confirmation of a diagnosis, trying a medication, or engaging in therapy, your plan suggests other things you could also be doing. When you ask, "What should I be doing now?" you're not starting from scratch. You can turn to your plan.

Your living treatment plan is also a communications tool. It keeps everyone involved in your care on the same page. They should all understand your treatment goals, symptoms, as well as which interventions have and haven't worked, and those still to be tried.

Plan, Meet Reality

You'll often hear your care providers refer to your treatment plan. A treatment plan describes your symptoms and diagnosis, along with a strategy to improve your mental health, such as using a certain medication. Often, these plans are written summaries created by your treatment provider after your first visit.

Unfortunately, these plans are frequently out of date as soon as they're written. You may not respond as hoped to a planned treatment. Choices that looked promising earlier now look iffy. Initial assumptions are rejected as your provider learns more about your experiences. Rather than providing ongoing guidance, your treatment plan is left to collect dust. We like to refer to these as dead treatment plans.

Without a plan, you're left with episodic care. Your appointments focus on short-term circumstances at the expense of the big picture. Sure, your treatment providers have some idea of where you're headed, however imprecise. Their chart notes are too detailed to help much. But with more patients and shorter and less frequent appointments, remembering the overall context and details of your plan gets harder. Increasingly, the focus is how you are feeling during the current visit. Next month it may be something completely different. Your treatment becomes reactive rather than proactive. You have no idea if you're making progress or if your current treatment is helping. It gets even worse if you have multiple treatment providers. Each one reacts to what they see each time they meet with you. And none of them may have any idea what your other treatment providers have just changed or what they'll do next.

Finding effective mental health treatment is a process of trial and error in which each trial can take weeks or months. You don't want to go down the wrong path, stay too long on an initially promising but ultimately unsuccessful treatment, or abandon what could have been an effective treatment too soon. Each misstep prolongs your return to wellness. Gaps in care such as waiting for specialists add delays and may derail your care entirely.

Creating the Plan

So, what does a living treatment plan look like? Check out Figure 14.1.

There's a lot going on here. We'll describe each piece in a moment, but you can see at a glance a variety of interventions and the results of trying them. Your treatment plan is a snapshot of your current situation, a record of what you've recently tried, and ideas you might try soon. As your treatment moves forward, your plan should adjust accordingly. To do that, it must be:

- quick and easy to create;
- quick and easy to modify;
- flexible enough to add all kinds of information;
- easy to show someone else; and
- compact enough to fit on one page (or screen).

Goals	improve concentration so able to go back to work within 3-6 months [Dec]

Symptoms	Differential diagnosis
• depressed mood [3] • anhedonia [8] • poor concentration and problem solving [8] • irritability [6]	• major depressive disorder • persistent depressive disorder • ~~bipolar disorder~~ • ? unspecified sleep disorder • ? mild cognitive impairment • ? adjustment disorder • ?? alcohol/substance use • ?? celiac disease

Current Interventions

TRY EFFEXOR
- plan: [Jul] 37.5mg x 2w, 75mg x 4w
  25% better after 75mg x 4w [mid-Aug]?
          - if so, continue increase...
  ⇒ side effect: excess sweating
      - try benztropine → worked!
      - eval: 25% benefit? → ✔
- continue increase 75mg x 2w to 225mg
  ⇒ side effect: sleep worse
      - change time of day take meds
      - add sleep med e.g. zopiclone?
  - eval: [Oct]

FIX LOW IRON [Aug: ferritin 17]

* Palafer (iron supplement)
    - recheck ferritin in 3mo [Nov]
    - check effect in 1mo [Sep]
- other supplement
? iron infusions

Potential Interventions

PHYSICAL HEALTH / LABS
- labs (common physical) ✔
  → ***LOW IRON**
    - repeat in 12mo [Aug]
? less common physical
? sleep apnea testing
?? MRI

PSYCHOTHERAPY
→ mindfulness meditation
? other psychotherapy

MEDICATIONS
antidepressants:
- ~~Zoloft (SSRI)~~ - nausea
* **EFFEXOR (SNRI)**
- Cymbalta (SNRI)
- Wellbutrin

LIFESTYLE FACTORS
→ reduce alcohol
? exercise more
~~less caffeine~~

VITAMINS / SUPPLEMENTS

OTHER

Figure 14.1: Sample living treatment plan.

The visual appearance of the plan isn't important. This example uses several spatially grouped textual outlines. It could just as well be represented as a mind map, a jumble of shapes and arrows, or a collection of scribbled sticky notes. It might use different colours, emojis, or other symbols to convey meaning. You can write it by hand in a notebook, use a word processor, drawing program, or outlining tool on a computer or tablet. The important thing is to use what works for you.

Portions of two alternative forms of the same plan are shown below. The one on the left shows all the interventions as a single outline, not broken down by categories. The flowchart-like one on the right uses different symbols to represent different types of elements.

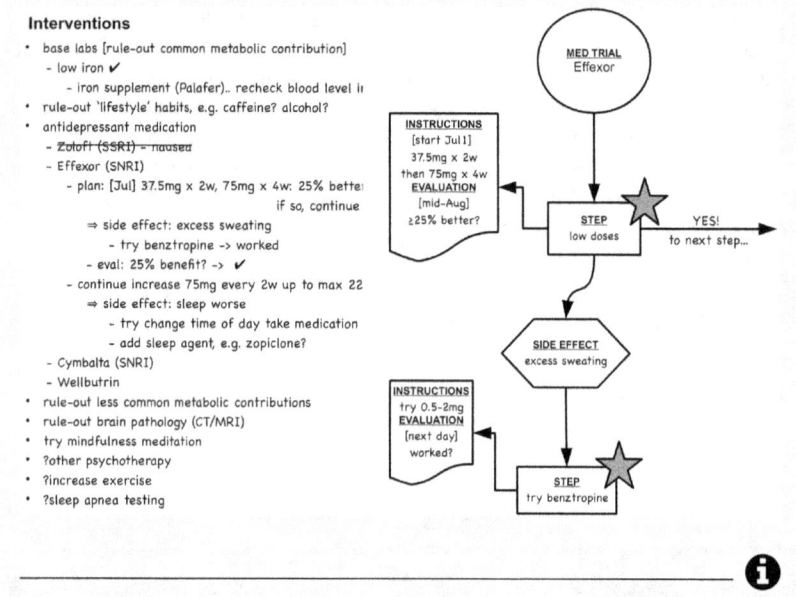

Components

We'll start by looking at the four main sections of the plan: symptoms, goals, diagnosis, and current and potential interventions.

You'll see shortly that the content of the plan can come from everyone on your treatment team, including yourself. Most of these sections may start out empty but will be filled out over time.

Symptoms

Your symptoms are the foundation for every other component of your living treatment plan. We covered labelling and measuring them in the *Describing Your Symptoms* chapter. Your living treatment plan identifies your main symptoms, as well as their severity or impact (the number in brackets).

Diagnoses

This section lists your diagnosis or diagnoses. Initially, this may be unclear. It may include possibilities to consider further. Over time, as you and your treatment providers work together, it will begin to solidify.

A list of diagnoses can inspire ideas for treatments and other interventions. Including possible diagnoses also reminds everyone to keep an open mind. If several treatment attempts have been unsuccessful, it may be worth revisiting your diagnosis.

This list of possible diagnoses is called the *differential diagnosis*. Adding a diagnosis to the differential is like asking, "Do I have X?" but not demanding an immediate answer. Think of it as a reminder to consider the diagnosis more closely in the future.

While most patients like to know their exact diagnosis, it's often not that clear-cut. You'll often see more tentative language, e.g., "rule out," "by history," and "possible." Confidence in your diagnosis can increase or come into doubt as you uncover more details about your illness. With enough evidence, it may be confirmed or ruled out.

Be open if your doctor suggests adding a diagnosis to consider even if it may feel uncomfortable. At the same time, you may have read about an illness that strikes a chord. Discuss with your doctor.

Goals

This section describes your treatment goals. These may be nothing more than "to not be sick anymore." But if you have many symptoms, goals help you prioritize what is most important to you. Often, your goals relate to how your overall quality of life has suffered due to your illness. What improvements do you most want to see? What activity would you like to start doing again? As with other parts of your plan, your goals may change over time.

A popular framework for goal setting is *SMART goals*. This acronym has several variations. Here is one:

- *Specific:* While "getting better" is a bit vague, "sleep through the night" is something more concrete to work on.
- *Measurable:* It should be easy to check if you've met your goal. For example, "at least six hours of sleep and felt well-rested in the morning, at least five days a week."
- *Achievable:* Be realistic. If you're sleeping two hours a night, "well-rested, optimal concentration and energy every day, without more sleep" sets you up for failure.
- *Relevant:* Goals should address aspects of your illness that most affect you. Don't focus on sleep if that's only a small part of what's bothering you.
- *Time-based:* Goals should have a timeframe for completion. This sets expectations and can impact the choice of treatments. If you want to sleep better by next week, you're going to need medications or supplements. If you have more time, other solutions such as therapy become possibilities.

Writing down explicit SMART goals helps ensure both you and your treatment providers have similar expectations. When goals are visible, it becomes easier to see when people have conflicting ideas. That can spark a valuable conversation that leads to a better, shared understanding. The alternative, where differences stay hidden, inevitably leads to frustration and people working at cross purposes.

Interventions

Rather than treatments, we'll speak more generally about interventions. An intervention can be a trial of a medication or a course of psychotherapy. It could be a lab test to rule out a vitamin deficiency or completion of a symptom scale to clarify a diagnosis. It may be doing more research to suggest alternative explanations for a problem.

Identifying potential interventions is a starting point. You also need to consider which are most likely to be effective at achieving your goals. These educated guesses help you choose which interventions to try next. You and your treatment providers should take into account not only clinical evidence, but also factors such as availability, cost, insurance coverage, and timeframe.

Potential interventions come from many places, including

- common (and less-common) treatments for your diagnosis;
- common (and less-common) treatments for particular symptoms;
- things that have worked well for you in the past;
- interventions suggested by other aspects of your medical history;
- things that have worked well for family members; and
- research.

The remainder of the book covers many different treatments and interventions. As you read further, consider which ones you might add to your treatment plan. Remember that finding the right treatments involves a certain amount of guesswork. Many ideal treatments (on paper) for your illness may not help you, while others will despite being intended for different uses. Better to include too many possibilities than too few. You're not committing to trying every single one of them.

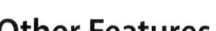

Other Features

There's more going on in our example living treatment plan than just lists of items in each section. We'll now draw your attention to several features of the plan that help to emphasize, differentiate, track, and manage each piece of your treatment. As you're reading, try to focus on what information each feature conveys and why it's important.

Ruled-Out Items

Your plan should highlight those things you're certain of versus those that are partially explored or future possibilities. Certainty may mean confirming a diagnosis, verifying you have a vitamin deficiency, or showing improvement on a medication. Whether noted with a check mark, gold star, or bright yellow highlighter, quickly picking out these items is important.

Less obviously, you should note interventions and other items that were once possibilities but are no longer. You found they either didn't apply or didn't work. For example, you'll notice several crossed-out items in the plan. You and your doctor initially considered several possible diagnoses, but after further discussion, you've ruled out a bipolar disorder. Here's another example. Using the medication Zoloft was a potential treatment option you considered, but after trying it, you found it made you too nauseous. Cross these out or move them to a "ruled-out" area but keep them somewhere.

Tracking things you've tried but that weren't helpful can serve as a reminder not to accidentally try them again later. Writing down what happened that made you change directions can also help. Review your medical records or try to recall treatments you've tried in the distant past as well.

Just because something didn't work at one point doesn't mean it won't work in the future. Your anxiety could have been too high to benefit from psychotherapy, or the particular therapist may have been a poor fit. You might not have tried a medication long enough or at an adequate dose. Look back at what didn't help you every so often. Has anything changed that might make revisiting an earlier intervention worthwhile?

Priority

Early in your treatment, there will be many more things you don't know than things you're confident about. But even in the beginning, you will consider some items in your plan more important than others. You might expect some interventions dealing with central issues to help, while others you may consider long shots. Making priority or importance explicit in your plan reminds you which items to pay more attention to and what steps you're likely to take next.

The example living treatment plan shows priority and importance in several different ways:

- The list of symptoms includes a number beside each to indicate its current severity or impact. A 1 is very minor, while a 10 is as bad as could be imagined.

- Ordering of lists can indicate likelihood or priority. For example, the list of diagnoses has the most likely ones at the top, with less likely ones further down.

- Different symbols can show priorities, such as one or more question marks (?) or asterisks (*). Some people use A, B, C or [H]igh, [M]edium, and [L]ow.

> Other common ways to show priority include changing the size of an item, the weight of the font, using different colours, adding boxes, lines, arrows, etc. Remember that the priority you assign to items may change over time.
>
>

Relationships

You'll notice that the Effexor intervention in the example is an outline several levels deep. This shows the relationships between different items. Why is an item in your plan? What are you taking that medication for? The outline puts each item in context. It reminds you how each part of your plan fits into the bigger picture. This global view keeps you from having tunnel vision and focusing too much on one small part of your treatment. Seeing everything is the reason we recommend your plan fit on one page or screen.

>
>
> The example treatment plan shows several different relationships.
>
> - Potential interventions are broken down into categories such as physical health, psychotherapy, etc. Medications currently contains one type: antidepressants. Antidepressants is itself a category with four particular examples: Zoloft, Effexor, Cymbalta, and Wellbutrin.
> - Within Effexor, you have two steps detailing how to start and then continue the medication.
> - Look at the sweating side effect. The solution below that is in response to the sweating, which in turn was in response to the Effexor.
>
> Why do these relationships matter? If you're having trouble dealing with the sweating side effect, they remind you that it's only a problem because of the Effexor. Does the Effexor even work well? If not, don't waste your time addressing its side effect.
>
>

Time

Another concept incorporated in a living treatment plan is time. Unlike an antibiotic that can kill off an infection in a few days, hardly anything in mental health happens quickly. Few people know what to expect from treatments including how long they take to work. Explicitly noting time in your treatment plans sets and communicates expectations. It reminds you to schedule evaluations to measure how well a treatment works. This helps avoid two common errors made treating mental illness. The first is spending far more time than needed on a remedy that isn't helping instead of stopping it and trying something else. The second is not spending enough time on a treatment to know if it will or won't work. You don't want to discard what could be an effective treatment without giving it a decent chance to work.

Notice the plan includes time as a duration, e.g., "recheck blood level in 3 mo" but also an absolute date, e.g., "1st week Sept." You might track those dates within your living treatment plan itself or on a separate calendar. Remember that as plans change, such as time spent dealing with a side effect before increasing a medication dose, you may need to adjust those dates.

Is time a significant consideration in your overall goals? Everyone would like to feel better sooner rather than later, but do you have a specific (and realistic) timeframe in mind? That affects the treatments you choose and whether you try more than one at a time. How long until you know if a treatment works? Some forms of psychotherapy work on very long timeframes, many months or years. Others can help in weeks. Some medications take effect in a matter of hours or days, but others can take weeks, after slowly increasing the dose. Knowing your goals helps your treatment providers suggest interventions that are appropriate for your desired timeframes and goals.

Summary

- A living treatment plan shows an overview of your current care, including your symptoms, goals, diagnoses, treatments, and other interventions. This includes potential treatments to be considered in the future.

- You update the plan as your situation changes, as you learn more about your illness, or discover potential treatments. It helps you see where you are now and plan for what might be next.

15

Using Your Plan

So now that you've seen all the different pieces of your living treatment plan and you understand why they're important, how do you use it?

This chapter answers that question in a few different ways. We'll first cover some basic principles for using your living treatment plan. Next, we'll look at various activities, such as starting a new treatment or evaluating a current one. We'll then show how time spent before, after, and between appointments can make the limited time available during appointments more productive and improve your overall treatment. Finally, we'll revisit some of the failure scenarios we described earlier to see how your living treatment plan corrects them.

As you read, keep in mind that reviewing and updating your plan is a great opportunity to involve family, friends, or other supports in your care.

The Basics

Your living treatment plan, whether ink on a page or pixels on a screen, is a road map. It helps you plan your mental health journey, and keep track of where you've been and where you're going. This isn't a solo journey. How you use your living treatment plan should reflect that.

Communication Tool

Your living treatment plan is first and foremost a communication tool. It's a picture of your treatment shared between you, your doctors and other treatment providers, and those family members or close friends you involve in your care. It makes explicit all the essential aspects of your current situation, goals, and treatment. This tool can help clarify any misunderstandings, especially when people involved have different expectations.

Ideally, your living treatment plan is an opportunity for collaboration between you and your care providers. If your treatment starts to deviate from the plan without warning, bring it up. It's important to raise issues proactively.

Your doctors or other treatment providers may choose to ignore your living treatment plan altogether when you try to share it with them. That's perfectly fine. It still helps for you to keep track of your treatment, clarify decisions, identify questions, and request advice from others. Your treatment provider may ignore the visible representation of your plan, but everyone still benefits as it helps you to actively contribute to your care.

Caretaker

Who actually makes changes to the living treatment plan document, in your notebook or electronic device?

We believe it's essential that you (possibly with help from family or friends), and not your doctor or another provider, be the caretaker of your living treatment plan. This helps you take ownership of your treatment and clarify and organize your care. It's especially important if several providers are involved. The onus is on you to update your plan.

Who Decides?

Next, consider a slightly trickier question. Who decides what to do at a specific time? Your living treatment plan contains elements such as diagnoses and interventions. Some items are for possible consideration in the future, some are more immediate. When it comes to choosing the treatments you'll actually pursue, who has the final say?

These decisions are ultimately up to both you and your treatment team. Your providers will help you do what they think is best in your situation. Your treatment plan helps you discuss your options with them, including positives and negatives from different peoples' perspectives. You may suggest options they would not have otherwise considered. But, at the end of the day, they're going to make decisions they're comfortable with.

You, on the other hand, have the right to consent (or not) to any particular treatment. That can admittedly be tricky, given the power differential, and often the scarcity of alternative treatment options. Your treatment plan can help you communicate your rationale and concerns about the alternatives. Ultimately, you decide if you want to proceed in a given direction. It's your life, after all.

Not every treatment needs someone else's approval or assistance for you to pursue it. You don't need anyone's permission to join a yoga class, take an over-the-counter supplement, or increase your exercise. Even so, include these in your plan. This keeps everyone aware of all your current interventions.

Activities

Let's look at the main activities your living treatment plan will be used for.

Sharing Your Plan

If your living treatment plan is primarily a communication tool, sharing it with others is essential.

When you meet a new provider, they want to know your concerns, what you've tried so far, and who else you're working with. Walking them through your plan can quickly get them up to speed. If they ask about why you're using a treatment, your plan should help you answer.

For current providers, use your plan to highlight what's changed since a previous visit. You may focus on small pieces, but the person you're talking with will view them in context, not in isolation.

Bring a copy of your plan to all appointments or when discussing your illness with family and friends. Sharing a single copy allows anyone to point to or otherwise emphasize elements of the plan. When physical circumstances don't allow, e.g., your therapist sits more than a few feet away from you, ensuring everyone has their own copy is a satisfactory alternative.

Goals, Symptoms, Diagnoses, and Interventions

Your plan contains concrete information such as what treatments or other interventions you're now engaged in. But it also includes the goals, symptoms, and even diagnoses that inform treatment decisions. Potential treatments to consider in the future are included for the same reason.

Add new elements to your plan to reflect a new understanding of your illness or for future consideration. Remove those that are no longer relevant. If a treatment didn't help, mark it as ruled out. Reprioritize elements so that the ones you feel are most relevant are up front and visible, while less important ones are examined only on a detailed read.

Where do all these elements come from? Your goals almost always come from you. Symptoms often come from you or those around you. Your care providers will ask you to track other symptoms they know are important. Your providers traditionally supply most diagnoses and treatment options.

But possible diagnoses and treatments might also come from you, based on things you've read, including the material on treatments in the rest of the book. Add them to your plan as a reminder to discuss them at a future visit.

Remember, the point of including possible diagnoses and treatments is to help make future decisions. If you're not familiar with something that's added, it's a cue to learn more to consider if or how it might apply to you.

Deciding What's Next

Your treatment plan will grow to include multiple possible interventions. Whether starting fresh or after stopping another treatment that didn't pan out, you need to decide what to try next.

You and your treatment providers can rank them by priority. Consider how likely they are to work (based on clinical evidence), but also how much time, effort, or other resources they require. Personal preferences and convenience are important, too. Having options in front of you is a good starting point. What to do next? Pick one of the higher-ranked items! You may favour one while a treatment provider prefers another, but a conversation around risks and benefits should highlight any tradeoffs.

Could you do more than one thing at a time? Sometimes it makes sense to try one thing before going on to the next. If you've decided to try an antidepressant and have five choices, don't start them all at once. Try one, and if it doesn't work, move on to the next.

At other times, it can make sense to try several things simultaneously. Let's say that your plan includes three possible treatments: take an iron supplement to correct a known deficiency, try an antidepressant, or start psychotherapy. You could try them one at a time. But it's also perfectly reasonable to pursue two or even all three at once.

> There is one downside to trying several things at once. If your symptoms improve, you can't be sure which of the things you've been doing made the difference. It could have been all of them, each contributing a bit, or just one—the others, were in some sense wasted efforts.
>
> Suppose all the improvements in the above scenario were from psychotherapy. But you don't know that, so you stay on the medication. That's one reason why people often try things sequentially. If you do try several things at once, add a reminder to your treatment plan to sort it out later with your treatment providers.

Starting a New Treatment

You've decided which treatment or intervention you're going to start next. If what you chose has been in your plan for a while, you had the opportunity to learn something about it. You'll undoubtedly still have questions, and your provider will want to emphasize certain things about the treatment.

When you begin anything new, it's important to set expectations. What's the plan for implementing the treatment, and what are your responsibilities? This may be straightforward if it means taking a pill or it may be more involved in some forms of therapy. What if something unexpected happens, e.g., side effects? Are there particular concerns to watch for?

You're trying this new treatment to see if it will work. What's the expected benefit if it does? How will you measure it? How long should it take to work? Is this a multi-step process? With many medications, for example, you start at a low dose, see if you can tolerate it, and gradually increase. You often won't see much benefit until you reach higher doses. Each step should still have a timeframe for evaluation in your living treatment plan.

You'll undoubtedly have more questions as you progress with the treatment or intervention. But in the beginning, you should broadly understand what the treatment looks like and what to expect.

Changing a Treatment

As you work through a treatment or intervention, sometimes you'll follow the plan that was sketched out when you first started it. Other times, changes will arise. With medications, for example, you may need to slow down or spread out increases in dosage. During therapy, you and your therapist might change course, bring in new concepts, spend more time exploring others, or add more sessions for another reason.

These types of changes are common. They often come about as everyone gains a better understanding of your illness and how to best tailor your treatment to you. However, be sure to update the timeframes and evaluation points in your treatment plan accordingly. When you adjust treatments, review your plan to see if these dates need to change. Make sure evaluation points are always scheduled for every intervention. The last thing you want is to make a change and then forget to check if that change, or the overall intervention, is actually helping you.

Sometimes changes will involve starting new treatments in conjunction with your current one, such as starting a new medication to resolve a side effect of another. Again, make sure you know what to expect and update your plan, including timeframes and evaluations.

Evaluating a Treatment

You've scheduled evaluations, but how do you check if a treatment is working? Go back to your symptoms! In the *Describing Your Symptoms* chapter, we explained severity (e.g., 1-10) as a way to measure them. We also talked about self-report rating scales and mood tracking apps. A before-and-after comparison of symptoms and severity should be part of each evaluation.

During treatment, watch for new symptoms or side effects emerging. Report them to your treatment provider and track them like your original symptoms. You can measure your progress on your own. This frees up your valuable appointment time for clarification and other activities. Your treatment providers will also ask questions and make observations as they determine if the intervention is helping or introducing new problems.

Be careful not to base your evaluations only on your symptoms if other factors are present. If the week leading up to an evaluation was unusually busy and you got some bad news, should you blame the drop in your mood on the treatment? Probably not. Speak up before someone changes your treatment without having all the facts.

A final question to consider: how good is good enough? Most guidelines recommend adjusting your treatment until all your symptoms are completely gone. Discuss this with your treatment providers after you're feeling a lot better. It's a decision based on your goals, your diagnosis, and the interventions you are using.

Appointments

You've just seen some of the most important activities that relate to your living treatment plan. How do you tie them all together? We'll look at that in the context of appointments with your treatment providers.

Most passive patients only think about their treatment and plan during all too brief appointments. But you're active in your care and guided by your living treatment plan. You spend time and effort before you arrive at your appointment and after you leave. That way, you get the very most out of each appointment. Let's see how.

Before

Prepare for your appointment by asking yourself a series of questions:

- What's new or what has changed since the last time you saw this provider? Has a different provider made changes to a treatment, suggested a diagnosis, or referred you for tests or other care?

- Have you added, removed, or reprioritized any elements in your plan?
- How are you doing overall? Consider updating the severity of symptoms in the plan. Any new problems or symptoms? Have there been any significant events or changes in your life since you last saw this treatment provider?
- Are you at an evaluation point? Check all dates in your plan for treatment steps or evaluation points. Often, appointments are scheduled to coincide with these. Can you provide a clear answer to whether the intervention is helping, or are you not sure?
- Do you have a course of action you'd like to propose at this appointment? A treatment change? A new alternative to consider? Something specific to focus on?

Take that information and make a concise list or set of notes to bring to your appointment. Your notes should help you summarize each point in a sentence or two. Make sure the most important points are upfront. You may be able to incorporate this into your living treatment plan or a copy. For example, you might use a highlighter to show which parts have changed or which you want to discuss in more detail.

During

All that preparation beforehand will pay off during your appointment. You shouldn't need to think on your feet about the basics. Be ready to share what you've prepared. Raise any significant changes or life events at the beginning.

If you're evaluating one step in an existing treatment, you'll have feedback to share, and your provider will probably have questions. They may review your diagnosis or discuss possibilities for future treatments. You may have things to contribute in these areas.

If decisions are needed, they're likely not coming out of the blue, but are already part of your living treatment plan. Regardless, make sure you know the risks, benefits, and alternatives. Speak up if you're uncomfortable or consider asking to postpone the decision to the next appointment so you can do some research in the meantime. Ask for recommended sources of information, if appropriate.

If making changes, ensure you know what to do and what to expect, including timeframes. Ask questions. Keep in mind what questions need answers now and which can wait until later.

After

Ideally, you (or someone you brought with you) were able to take quick notes during the appointment itself. Otherwise, it's time for a memory dump immediately after your appointment. Spend a few minutes in the waiting room or in your car before driving off, but don't wait until hours later.

Preferably sooner rather than later, turn your quick notes into something you'll be able to understand later, filling in details. If you brought someone with you, doing it together will help clarify things. If you've got questions as you go, write them down. You may be able to find the answers yourself or you may need to check with your treatment provider, either at the next appointment or even before.

When you have time, update your living treatment plan with any changes or new information. If changes are made that affect other pieces of the plan, such as dates, adjust them as necessary.

Between

In the time between appointments, you can do a lot of housekeeping work with your living treatment plan. Keep your plan tidy and relevant. Scan through it once in a while. Is everything up to date? Are priorities for each item current? Do diagnoses and interventions reflect everyone's latest insights? Did anyone suggest possible diagnoses or interventions you should add to the plan? Are some things so unlikely you can remove them from the plan altogether? When will you next be evaluating each current intervention? Is anything overdue? Things such as repeating labs, which have timeframes of many months, often slip. Have you updated the severity of your symptoms in the plan recently?

Beyond housekeeping, there may be some deep work that can significantly move your plan forward. Just like a series of experiments, your treatment plan evolves by eliminating unknowns. Whether a treatment works or not is only one part of this. Are there elements of your plan that could benefit from further reading or research? The *Paging Dr. Google* chapter can help with this. If some items in the plan need further investigation, is there anything you can do? If it's a possible diagnosis, are there symptom self-report scales or other reading you could do that might help your providers? Do you have old medical records that might help? If you are considering an intervention, do you understand it well enough to see how it could fit into your plan? What are its good and bad points from your perspective?

Before and After

In the *Working with Your Family Doctor* chapter, we gave examples showing how a family doctor's challenges can affect your treatment. Let's revisit some of them here and see what difference a living treatment plan makes.

Identifying Alternatives

> Along with your low mood, you mention being always tired and having memory problems. Your doctor prescribes you an antidepressant and, two months later, a different one—neither help. What they didn't do is check your iron level and find an easily fixed deficiency that can quickly improve your energy and memory.

Your doctor identified only a single treatment option (antidepressant medication). When it didn't work, they tried a variation of the same thing. Even early on, the treatment plan should have identified other options. Those could include blood work to look for a metabolic cause of your symptoms. These tests are cheap and fast. There's no reason not to do them before or at the same time as trying a medication. Other options you might add to the plan, even if not done immediately, would be diagnostic imaging, cognitive testing, or psychotherapy.

Living treatment plans identify alternatives, so you avoid tunnel vision. They help break out of the one-thing-at-a-time mindset that episodic care encourages.

Sharing Expectations

> Your doctor tries you on an antidepressant and books a follow-up in three weeks. At that visit, you complain of nausea and brain fog. They stop the antidepressant due to side effects. Because it's such a short appointment, you do not discuss that you only filled the prescription three days ago due to your anxiety. You miss out on a medication that could have worked very well once your system got used to it.

Here, a treatment is being eliminated from the plan prematurely. Chalk this up to poor communication. The doctor thinks you've been on the medication for three weeks. You didn't know that some side effects go away with time and didn't think to mention you just filled the prescription. One key aspect of good treatment plans is that they explicitly include the length of time before evaluating treatments. This helps avoid these miscommunications.

Closing Gaps

> *Your family doctor refers you to a local mental health clinic. They complete a quick intake appointment and put you in an eight-week mindfulness course. While interesting, it doesn't help address your particular mental health symptoms. Your family doctor assumes your mental health concerns were taken care of at the clinic. They don't pursue any other possible avenues of treatment.*

Several things are happening. First, the clinic created their own (traditional) treatment plan at the intake: "do mindfulness course." It describes what they think is the most promising option based on what they know at the start. There's no evaluation or other treatment alternative.

Your doctor thinks they've entirely handed off your care to the clinic. The clinic is worrying about the mindfulness course. Nobody is considering any alternatives. A single, comprehensive living treatment plan shared by your doctor, the clinic, and you would ensure that every intervention (e.g., "send to mental health clinic") has both a timeline and an evaluation phase. Your doctor would find out if your symptoms haven't improved and why, leading to a new intervention.

Stay Moving

> *They refer you to a psychiatrist with a 12- to 18-month waiting list. When asked what to do in the meantime, they shrug and say, "I've already referred you to someone, what more do you want?"*

Again, a good plan highlights alternatives, which may not need to take place one after the other. There's no reason not to try other treatments while you are waiting to see a psychiatrist. In the meantime, what worked and what didn't would be passed on to the psychiatrist.

Summary

- You're in charge of your living treatment plan document, but decision making about treatments is shared between you and your treatment providers.
- Preparing for your appointments with treatment providers helps you get the most out of the limited time you have available with them during appointments.
- The time between appointments can be used to both update and organize your living treatment plan, and for reading, research, and other activities to significantly enhance your overall treatment.

Part III

Treatments

16

So Many Choices!

So far, you've learned a great deal about how to improve the quality of your mental health care: from setting expectations, to doing research, to improving your relationship and communication with your treatment providers. You've learned how to use your living treatment plan to avoid the many pitfalls that can so easily derail care.

You have the tools to master the process and logistics. It's now time to explore the broad range of treatments and interventions available. What do they do? How do they work? What problems can each help with? How do you even begin to choose the treatments that are right for you? The remainder of the book tackles these questions.

There is a massive amount of material here and we're only covering it in summary form. The sheer number of interventions available to treat mental illness creates a big challenge.[1] Patients, family doctors, psychiatrists, psychologists, and counsellors—everyone finds it hard to keep track. New treatments and new ways of understanding old treatments are constantly appearing. It can be overwhelming. The good news is that, with so many more treatments, the chances of finding an effective one for you are higher than ever before.

If there's one message we hope you've heard loud and clear, it's that everyone is different. Your experience with mental illness is different from everyone else's. Discovering the interventions that are relevant to and will work for you is very personal. You won't find recipes here saying, "If you have depression, do X." The interventions you incorporate into your living treatment plan will be those that make sense for you.

You'll learn the importance of matching symptoms, causes, and treatments. The best treatment won't help if it doesn't address the causes underlying your illness. There may be no way to identify these causes—one of the reasons trial and error is needed. You'll find the most natural, holistic treatments have far more in common with hardcore pharmaceuticals than you'd imagine. In mental health, you can accomplish the same thing in many different ways. There's no magic here.

So, what sorts of interventions will we cover? We'll start by looking at your physical health, which is deeply intertwined with your mental health. You'll learn how some physical illnesses can bring on mental health symptoms or even increase the chance of developing a mental illness. We'll look at various substances in your body such as vitamins and minerals that impact your mental health. We'll discuss how to ensure deficiencies aren't worsening your symptoms.

Next, we'll look at lifestyle factors, including diet, exercise, sleep, alcohol, caffeine, tobacco, cannabis, and illicit drugs. We'll explore the positive and negative effects these can have on your mental health. We'll talk about vitamins, supplements, and other natural treatments used for mental health. We'll try to separate fact from fiction.

We'll then turn to the vast and varied collection of psychotherapies. These can have different roles in treatment. We'll introduce the many different professionals who work in the field and suggest some approaches to find someone who's right for you. We'll talk about therapies that can provide practical, day-to-day support. We'll also examine evidence-based psychotherapies, some widely applicable, some focused on particular mental illnesses. We'll look at the challenges often associated with accessing individual or group therapy. We'll also cover self-help and other resources that provide alternative ways to learn many techniques taught in therapy.

The remaining chapters deal with psychotropic medications, i.e., those for mental health, including antidepressants, mood stabilizers, and others. As compared to other mental health treatments, medications are more complicated and misunderstood. Given that, we'll devote plenty of attention to the fundamentals. You'll learn how they work, how they are chosen, how they can (and cannot) help, and why they're frequently used. We fully appreciate that medications aren't for everyone. We hope you can suspend any preconceived notions and approach this material with an open mind. We want you to make well-informed decisions about whether medications, like any other treatments, have a place in your living treatment plan.

We'll look in some detail at antidepressants, which are the most frequently prescribed psychotropic medications. Building on that material, we'll cover other categories of medications as well. We'll talk about how medications are properly used, what to expect from them, how long they'll take to work, and so on. We'll discuss the smart way to try medications and how to avoid abandoning them prematurely. We'll review managing side effects and special situations such as pregnancy.

Along the way, we'll show you the common errors that we see all the time. Better you learn from other peoples' mistakes than your own.

No Silver Bullet

If you read the in-depth article on our website that was mentioned under *Lies, Damn Lies, and Evidence* (in *Paging Dr. Google*), you know what we're going to say here. For everyone else, pay attention!

> *No matter how many people say that a specific treatment will solve your particular problem, don't believe them. Mental illness and its treatments are far too varied and affected by far too many factors. Current science can point you in the right direction but can't make predictions. All the studies and evidence in the world can't tell you what treatment will definitely work for you. Evidence can help guide your predictions. Trial and error, possibly lengthy, will almost certainly be needed to fully treat your illness.*

Getting Started

The remaining chapters describe many different interventions. How do you begin to choose which belong in your living treatment plan? If you're not sure, here's one approach to consider:

1. First, we're going to assume that you have at least a tentative diagnosis from your doctor or another mental health professional. If not, start there. We'll also assume you've started your living treatment plan in your notebook or electronic gizmo. You're ready to start trying things.

2. Next, make sure to read the following chapter, *Just Enough Neuroscience*. You'll need this to understand both what various treatments can do and what they can't do. This will also help you compare different treatments. It will save you from trying five similar solutions for a single problem. Instead, you could be trying a range of things, increasing the chances of finding those that work.

3. Read the chapter *Your Physical Health,* and then go see your doctor. Are there medical explanations for your symptoms that should be considered? A simple blood test could identify a problem with a quick solution. Better to start there rather than spending months in therapy or taking antidepressants with limited benefit.

4. Look through the *Lifestyle Factors* chapter. Are you unknowingly doing anything that might be making your mental health symptoms worse? Is there something you are able and willing to change that might help? Will any of these lifestyle factors affect how likely other treatments are to work?

5. Skim the chapters on the other treatments and add ideas that seem relevant to your living treatment plan. You're not committing to them now. You're highlighting them so you can read a bit more and possibly raise them with your care providers. As you're skimming, ask yourself some questions. Does this treatment seem like it might be applicable or relevant to your situation? Might it be available to you? Is this something you might be interested in trying?

Summary

- There are an incredible number of different treatments for mental illness. The difficult part is identifying the ones right for you. It's not possible to predict what will work, and so, trial and error is involved.

- Everyone is different. Because a treatment worked for someone you know does not mean it will work for you, even if you have the same illness or your symptoms seem very similar. Treatments have to match the underlying causes of your illness, which may not be possible to determine.

17

Just Enough Neuroscience

Neuroscience is the study of the brain and nervous system. The general overview here will give you a basic understanding of how mental health interventions affect your thoughts and emotions. It's not as simple as implied by common phrases such as "chemical imbalances" or "you don't have enough serotonin." Knowing this, you'll be better able to contribute to your care and treatment plan. Otherwise, you're more likely to make treatment decisions based on emotion instead of logic. Don't worry. We're not talking PhD material here. We'll keep this as painless as possible.

The Big Picture

Your brain consists of nerve cells called neurons, each connected to other neurons, creating a network like that shown in Figure 17.1. Well, it's a bit bigger. In reality, your brain has upwards of 80 billion neurons, each with up to 1,500 connections to other neurons.

Your brain constantly sends signals over this network, from one neuron to the next. When these signals reach different parts of your brain, they cause things to happen, e.g,. your left foot moves forward. Every thought, feeling, sensation, or memory is a result of signals sent between neurons.

Your brain continuously creates new connections between neurons. It also creates new neurons, though not as often as it makes new connections. When you learn, your brain is making these new connections.

Your entire personality, behaviour, and consciousness emerges based on the entire pattern of connections between the billions of neurons in your brain. It's similar to how a complex computer program emerges when millions of 1s and 0s are placed in the right order.

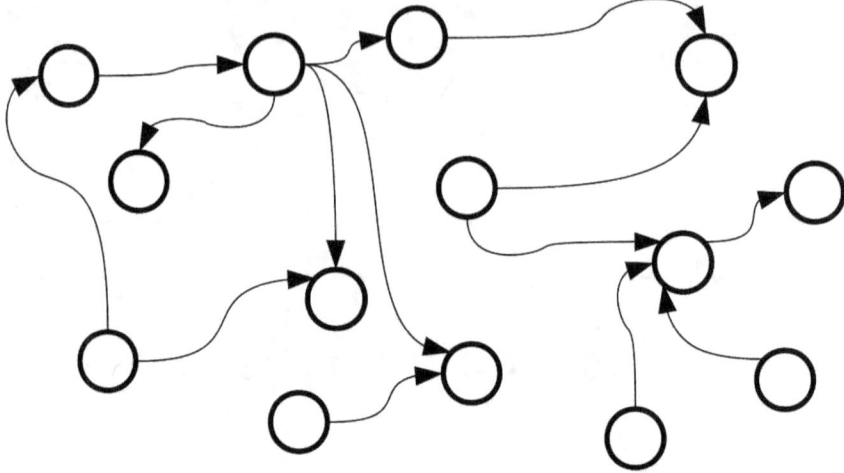

Figure 17.1: A network of interconnected neurons.

Neurons and Signals

Neurons receive signals from other neurons. Based on the signals it receives, each neuron turns on or off like a switch. When it's on, it sends signals to the neurons it is connected to. When it's off, no signals are sent. Each neuron contains a part to receive signals, a part that (among other things) decides whether to turn itself on or off, and a part that transmits signals. This is conceptually illustrated in Figure 17.2.

Decision Time

Pretend you're a neuron. How do you decide whether to turn on or off? The first thing to know is that there are two basic types of signals, excitatory (on) and inhibitory (off). At any given time, some of the hundreds of neurons connected to you have sent you an excitatory signal, some an inhibitory signal, and some no signal at all.

If you receive more excitatory signals than inhibitory signals, you'll be on. If there are more inhibitory signals, you'll be off. This process is called summation (think of every excitatory signal as a +1, every inhibitory signal as a -1, and add them up; if the sum is more than 0, the neuron is on).

If you are on, you transmit signals to all the neurons you're connected to. Other neurons are connected to different neurons than you are and receive signals from them. Each neuron reacts differently than every other neuron because it has a unique set of connections.

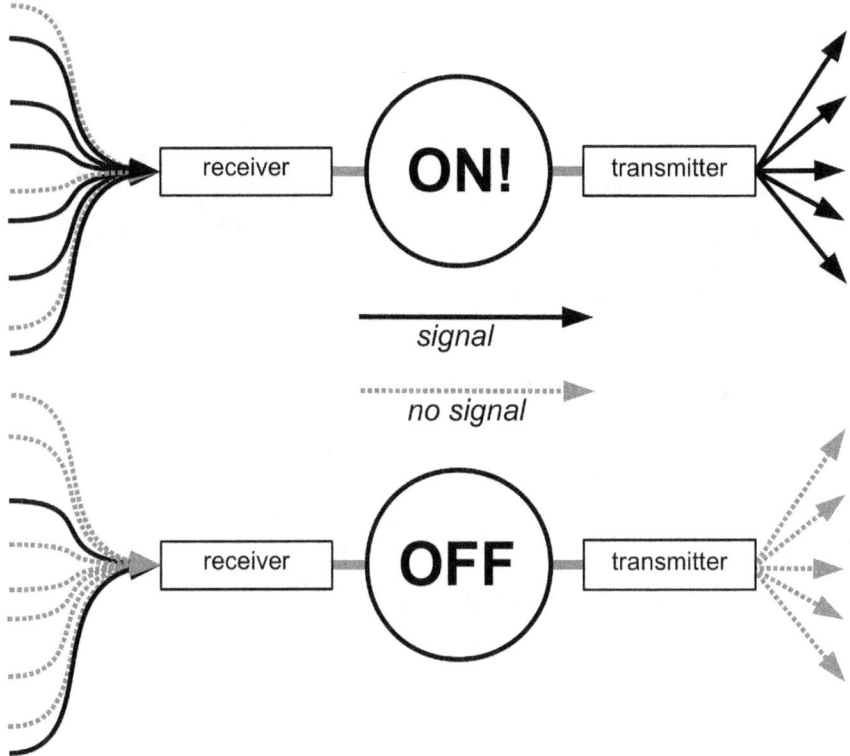

Figure 17.2: Depending on the signals it receives, a neuron can be on (top) or off (bottom).

Connecting Neurons

So far, we've treated neurons as if they were nice compact shapes, where the transmitting part of one is connected to the receiving part of another as if they're wired together. The two kinds of signals are like two different strength electrical currents. That's not exactly true.

For starters, neurons aren't compact, simple shapes. Instead, they look more like the gangly structure shown in Figure 17.3. Signals are received from other neurons by dendrites. The cell body processes the signals as we just described. Any outgoing signals are sent along the axon, where they are passed from an axon terminal to the dendrites of another neuron.

Second, neurons aren't physically connected to one another. There's a small space, called a synapse, between the axon terminal of one and the dendrites of another. To transmit a signal, a neuron must bridge that synapse. It does this by releasing chemicals, called neurotransmitters, that drift around in the synapse, as shown in Figure 17.4.

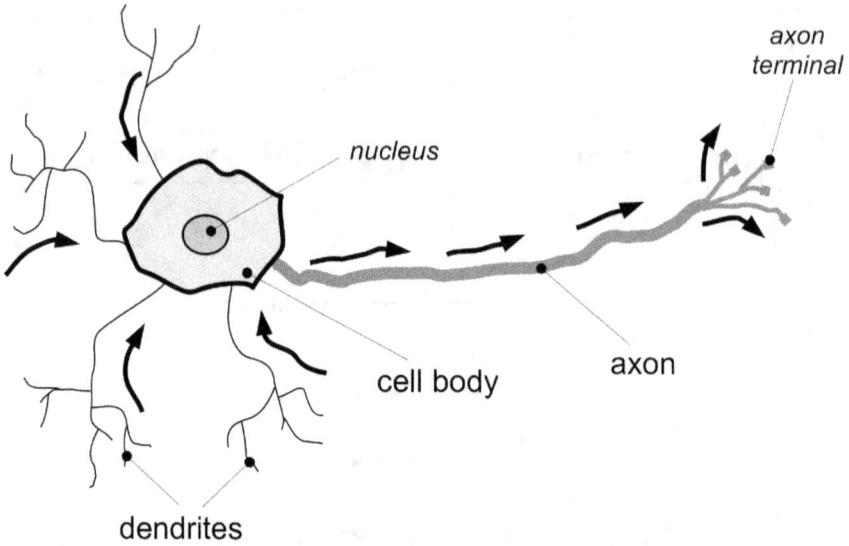

Figure 17.3: Structure of a neuron. Arrows show the flow of signals.

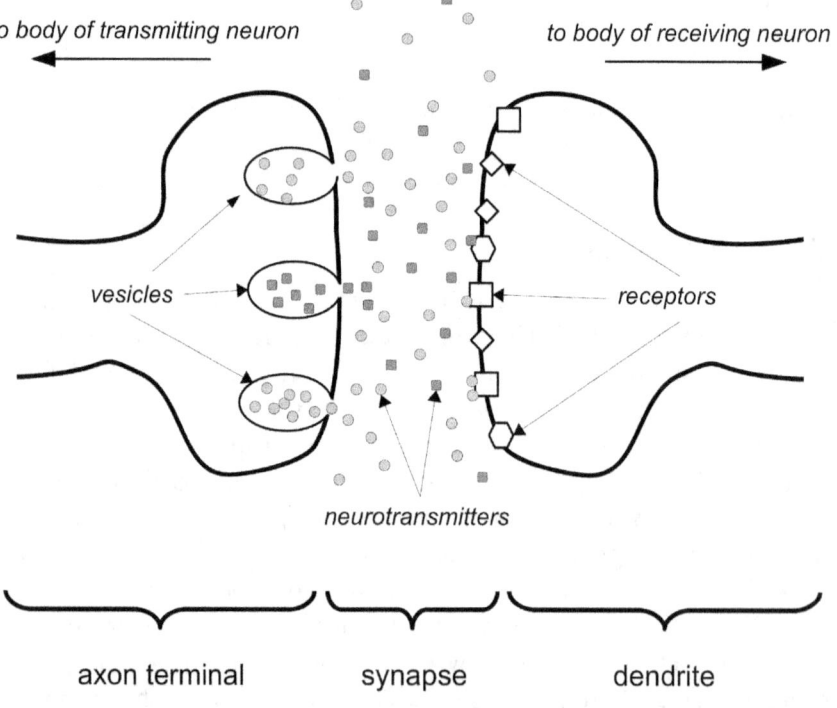

Figure 17.4: Signals being passed across a synapse using neurotransmitters.

Across the synapse and attached to the dendrite, there are objects called receptors. When a neurotransmitter drifts close to a receptor, the receptor grabs it and holds on. While it's holding the neurotransmitter, the signal has been sent (it now registers as +1 or -1 to the receiving neuron).

More on Neurotransmitters

The axon of each neuron stores neurotransmitters to be released when the neuron is on. They are stored in sacs called vesicles. Releasing the neurotransmitters is like opening a door between a vesicle and the synapse.

Neurons also create neurotransmitters in the first place, from smaller building blocks called precursors. These are either brought in from outside the neuron or are byproducts of other things going on in the neuron.

There are more than 100 types of neurotransmitters, both excitatory and inhibitory. The most important ones affecting mental health are *serotonin, norepinephrine, dopamine,* and *gamma-aminobutyric acid (GABA)*.

More on Receptors

Just as there are different neurotransmitters, there are different receptors. Each accepts only one type of neurotransmitter. Usually, there are several types of receptors for each neurotransmitter. The dendrites of a neuron can have many receptors (all the same or of different types).

What happens to a neurotransmitter after it is grabbed by a receptor? The receptor holds onto it for some length of time (dependent on the type of receptor) and then releases it back into the synapse.

Receptors grab neurotransmitters only when they drift close by. There's no guarantee a neurotransmitter will find a receptor. But the more neurotransmitters in the synapse, the more likely a receptor will grab one.

Cleanup

Neurotransmitters don't drift around the synapse forever. If they did, signals would keep being sent over and over. Three things happen to reduce the number of neurotransmitters in the synapse. First, they can drift away from the synapse, to be absorbed by other cells in the nervous system. They can be broken down by enzymes. Finally, they can be reabsorbed by the axon, called reuptake. This makes them available to be released again in the future.

Effects of Treatments

Armed with your newfound knowledge of neuroscience, you may be asking: how is this related to mental health treatments? Here's a quick preview.

We started off saying that feelings (and everything else) are a result of signals travelling between neurons. To greatly simplify, the greater the number of signals sent through the network by, for example, the neurotransmitter serotonin, the happier we feel. More signals mean that more serotonin receptors are activated. The more the merrier, literally!

Treatments take advantage of this by doing one or more of these things:

- Ensuring enough serotonin or its precursors (i.e., nutrients) are available. Signals can't be steadily sent if you're deficient. However, boosting beyond normal levels won't help. Neurons will only create, store, and release as much serotonin as they need.
- Stimulating the axon to release more neurotransmitters when activated. This is akin to opening the vesicle door wider. The more neurotransmitters in the synapse, the more likely they'll find a receptor.
- Adding another chemical that looks like serotonin into the synapse. This tricks receptors into grabbing it and activating as if it were serotonin.
- Slowing the reuptake of serotonin from the synapse back into the axon, so more remains in the synapse longer.

Different treatments can affect serotonin and other neurotransmitters via different mechanisms. If two treatments use the same mechanisms to affect the same neurotransmitters, they'll give similar results. That's true even if one is a pharmaceutical and another is a natural supplement.

> ### *Summary*
> - Thoughts, emotions and behaviours emerge from signals sent between neurons. Neurons are either on, at which time they send signals, or off. Changes in the connections between neurons occur with learning.
> - Signals are sent by neurotransmitters such as serotonin, norepinephrine, dopamine, and GABA through the synapse between neurons and grabbed by receptors. These determine if the neuron is on or off.
> - Treatments affect whether neurotransmitters are successfully sent across the synapse. They can change the number of neurotransmitters available, change how long they remain in the synapse, or block receptors.

18

Physical Illness

It shouldn't come as a shock that your physical and mental health are connected. But you may be surprised just how interconnected they actually are.

If something is wrong in your brain, it makes sense that it could affect your mood and behaviour. Yet, the connections go far deeper than that. If you have some physical illnesses, such as coronary artery disease, you're far more likely to develop mental health issues such as depression and anxiety. It works the other way too. Untreated mental health issues greatly increase your chances of developing certain physical illnesses. They can also lead to poorer outcomes of physical illness. It's one of the many reasons why treating mental illness is so important.

Why do we say addressing physical illness is a mental health treatment? Quite simply, illness may contribute to or cause your mental health symptoms. Dealing with physical health problems may reduce or eliminate mental health problems.

Needless to say, this chapter may not be the gentlest read for hypochondriacs. It's also not great if you avoid doctors in case they "find something." Yet, it's still tame compared with an internet search on any symptom you care to mention. We are not suggesting you test for any physical illness that could possibly cause a symptom. Based on your history, physical and mental health symptoms, and your response to treatment, your doctor can judge what to look at further.

Physical Illness Impacts Mental Health

If you're having new mental health symptoms, could a physical health issue be contributing? It's one of the first things you and your mental health providers should think about. This is particularly true if this is your first experience with mental health symptoms and no obvious stressful events have occurred recently.

Assuming that no physical factors are contributing to your symptoms is a lost opportunity at best. At worst it could be dangerous. Treating a physical illness with antidepressants or psychotherapy will likely fail. Dulling your symptoms with benzodiazepines or antipsychotics may help in the short term. However, unless your physical illness gets better on its own, they won't help you in the long run. Sometimes mental health symptoms are the first signs of a physical illness. Identifying and treating a physical illness early is easier than waiting until other symptoms develop.

If you have long-term, chronic physical health conditions such as diabetes or cardiovascular disease, you're at higher risk of developing mental illness. This, in turn, can worsen your physical illness. Without prompt attention, a devastating negative feedback loop can develop.

Illnesses With Mental Health Symptoms

Sometimes the first signs of a physical illness are what appear to be purely mental health symptoms. Someone with a brain tumour may first develop changes in mood or energy, hallucinations or other psychosis, or even drastic personality changes. It's easy to understand why since the physical illness directly affects the brain.

Indirectly, deficiencies in iron or other vitamins and minerals can cause mood swings, decreased energy, and poor memory and concentration. We'll closely examine these deficiencies in the next chapter. Hormone changes can also cause mental health issues. Illnesses such as diabetes, polycystic ovarian syndrome, Addison's disease, and some cancers all affect hormones, as do normal fluctuations associated with menstruation, pregnancy, and perimenopause in women.

Treatments

If physical health problems can lead to mental health symptoms, so can many treatments for those physical health problems. All medications and natural supplements have possible side effects, including mental health side effects. One broad study[1] found that 37% of participants who reported depression used at least one medication that listed depression as a side effect. Here are just a few examples of such medications:

- Accutane (acne);
- Keppra (anticonvulsant for epilepsy);

- Chantix/Champix (stop smoking);
- Estrogen (menopause, osteoporosis, birth control); and
- Interferon (hepatitis, some cancers).

The following medications often cause anxiety as a side effect:
- Prednisone and other corticosteroids (allergies, asthma, inflammation);
- Albuterol and other bronchodilators (asthma, COPD);
- Zyban/Wellbutrin (stop smoking, depression); and
- Antihistamines (high dose for allergies).

Increased Risk

Chronic physical illness increases the risk of mental health problems over time. The increased risk can be related to biological changes from illness, chronic pain, and treatments for the illness itself. There are many psychosocial issues as well. Physical illness can lead to lifestyle changes or disability, and may affect finances or relationships. It can raise challenging existential questions. You may experience grief and loss over dreams you can't achieve because of poor health. The increased risk of mental illness is substantial.[2] Here are a few examples:

- People with chronic physical conditions have double the risk of experiencing a mood or anxiety disorder versus those without a chronic physical condition.
- People with heart disease are three times more likely to develop depression than people without.
- Concerning respiratory disorders, around 75% of people with severe COPD (chronic obstructive pulmonary disease) have depression or anxiety. Those with asthma have a significantly increased likelihood of anxiety or panic.

People with chronic physical illness who develop a mental illness have worse outcomes. The costs to the health system of their treatment—for their physical illness alone—are much higher. They are less compliant with treatment recommendations and more likely to develop poor habits in areas such as diet, exercise, sleep and substance use, that will affect their physical health.

Impact on Treatment

Physical illness also affects how mental illness is treated, even if the two are entirely unrelated. Treatments for mental illness need to factor in any physical illness. Here is why:

- Physical illness can leave you more prone to vitamin and mineral deficiencies. These can prevent antidepressants from working.
- Some medications and supplements for mental illness are not safe to use if you have certain physical illnesses.
- Medications for mental health can worsen physical health symptoms. Many also interact with the medications being used to treat those physical conditions.

Mental Illness Impacts Physical Health

Don't think that the effects of physical illness on mental health are a one-way street. Mental illness also affects physical illness in very similar ways.

Symptoms

When feeling mentally unwell, you may also have physical symptoms. These are also known as somatic symptoms, i.e., those affecting the body. Some examples are

- pain;
- nausea;
- lack of energy;
- agitation and restlessness;
- changes in appetite and weight; and
- dizziness.

People who are less comfortable with expressing emotion often have more somatic complaints. Members of certain cultures tend to express emotions somatically. Men do this far more often than women.

Treatments

As in all areas of medicine, medications for mental illness often produce physical side effects. They target neurotransmitters in the brain but affect those in the body as well. They can potentially cause nausea, headache, tremor, dizziness, heart rate or blood pressure changes, skin reactions, and many more conditions.

Taken long-term, some of these medications can pose additional risks. These may include obesity, increased cholesterol, changes in heart rhythm, kidney failure, osteoporosis, and other physical changes. Periodic monitoring can detect changes before they become problems.

Increased Risk

Just as having a physical illness increases the likelihood of developing a mental illness, having a mental illness increases the risk of developing a physical illness. Here are a few examples:

- Those who have symptoms of depression have triple the number of chronic physical health conditions compared to the general population.
- Women with depression are 80% more likely to experience heart disease than women without depression.
- People with some mental illnesses have as much as a three times increased risk of a stroke.
- There are established connections between mental illness and increased inflammation, a decreased immune system, and increased digestive distress.

There is another, more insidious impact of mental illness on your physical health to be aware of. People with a mental illness are much more likely to have their physical complaints not taken as seriously as people without mental illness. Too many people are inclined to believe "it's all in your head" or at least that things aren't as bad as you're describing. It's a phenomenon known as *diagnostic overshadowing* and it can have very serious consequences. This attitude is regrettably common in the general population. Far too many healthcare practitioners are also guilty of this.[3]

Your Role

We hope you better appreciate the close interconnection between mental and physical illness. It's one reason we feel so strongly that medical doctors should play a role in your mental health.

You may not follow the medical model or perhaps you favour alternative treatments. However, if you're not improving, we'd encourage you to expand your perspective. Make sure there's not a physical health problem contributing. Use your living treatment plan to prevent tunnel vision, consider alternatives, and reevaluate your treatments.

The intersection of physical and mental health is a potential trouble spot in your care. Professionals working on the physical or mental health side of the divide are often unaware of what's happening on the other side. It's your responsibility to bridge this gap. If you're proceeding with therapy, talk to your doctor about whether a physical illness could be having an effect. Make sure they know your full health history, even if you think parts don't matter. If you have multiple professionals involved in your mental health care, it's up to you to let each one know what the others are up to.

> ### Summary
>
> - Physical and mental illness are deeply intertwined. People with certain physical illnesses are more likely to develop certain mental illnesses. Treating a physical illness can be more complicated and may be less likely to succeed when a mental illness is present. The reverse is also true.
>
> - The first signs of some physical illnesses can be mental health symptoms. Brain tumours and some vitamin deficiencies are examples. Many medications for physical illnesses also have mental health symptoms as side effects. Sometimes mental health problems can appear as physical or somatic symptoms.
>
> - Even if you don't plan on pursuing medical treatments such as antidepressants for your mental health concerns, see a doctor to make sure there's not an obvious physical health cause.

19

Lab Investigations

The previous chapter discussed the link between physical and mental illness. Here, we'll describe tests for common problems affecting mental health. No, there is not a blood test to diagnose mental illness. But when you first talk to a doctor, don't be surprised if they reach for a lab requisition form rather than a prescription pad.

We don't recommend you be tested for everything imaginable. That would be a spectacular waste of resources. At the same time, you shouldn't be left unable to function for years because someone didn't order an inexpensive blood test. One of the best ways to avoid unnecessary testing is knowing what's already been tested. If you have a regular family doctor, your lab results are probably in their Electronic Medical Record (EMR) system. But, that doesn't mean that other doctors know about them.[1]

Most family doctors send recent lab test results to specialists when you are referred, but not always. They may also neglect to send tests done later. If you've had recent tests, make sure everyone involved in your care knows about it. The best way is to get copies of your own results. You may be able to see your results online or ask the lab or your doctor for a copy. This also helps if you see multiple doctors. It can save a lot of hassle, money, and time.

Iron

Low iron can cause several symptoms also found in those with depression. These include fatigue, decreased energy, memory problems, and poor concentration. It can cause restless legs often thought to be solely due to medication. Low iron can also affect your treatment. It reduces the effectiveness of psychotropic medications, limits your exercise capacity, and more.

Routine blood work will check your hemoglobin, the iron-rich component of your blood. That test detects only very low iron. However, even a moderate deficiency can impact mental health. A better measure is serum ferritin (stored iron). Labs consider normal ferritin to be about 15–270 µg/l. However, if you have mental health concerns, 15 is too low. It should be higher, preferably at least 50.

We've seen many people whose "depression" disappears after treating their iron deficiency. This is one of the few no-brainer fixes. Also, keep in mind that your iron levels can change over time. Has your energy decreased or your concentration worsened, for no apparent reason? Has a long-term medication become less effective or "pooped out" altogether? Ask your doctor to recheck your ferritin before making other changes.

The test for serum ferritin indicates how much iron is stored in your blood outside your red blood cells. A routine complete blood count (CBC) measures hemoglobin, the iron inside your red blood cells. You can have normal hemoglobin but low ferritin.

Iron stores help with many things, including building neurotransmitters. Too little iron means too few neurotransmitters. Trying to fix depressive symptoms brought on by low iron with treatments such as antidepressants won't work. Low iron can impair energy, concentration, and memory.

Low iron may mean you don't get enough in your diet, you may absorb it poorly, or you may have heavy bleeding or another illness. Changes in diet, supplements, or working with your doctor to deal with physical illnesses can help.

Vitamin B12

If iron deficiency is the number one missed opportunity for a quick fix, low vitamin B12 runs a close second. Like iron, B12 is needed to make red blood cells, as well as for the proper operation of the nervous system. A severe deficiency can cause similar problems: weakness, fatigue, numbness, tremor, depression, anxiety, confusion, and poor memory.

Low B12 can result from inadequate dietary intake. As B12 is not naturally found in plant foods, vegans require fortified foods or supplements. Absorption problems can also reduce B12 levels. The ability to absorb vitamin B12 decreases with age, so this affects seniors more frequently. Many of the cognitive symptoms of B12 deficiency mimic those of early-stage dementia. A missed blood test can result in unnecessary concern.

Again, the normal reference range for vitamin B12 is a bit too low, typically around 150–655 pmol/l. Studies have shown that for those experiencing mental health symptoms, the minimum level should be higher—at least 240 pmol/l. A vitamin B12 deficiency can be easily missed. For those with very low B12, recovery after starting oral supplements or a quick injection can be dramatic.

Like iron, B12 is needed to create neurotransmitters such as serotonin, norepinephrine, dopamine, and GABA. It also serves another important function in the nervous system, producing myelin. Myelin is an insulating layer that surrounds the long axons of nerves, acting like insulation around an electrical wire. A lack of myelin reduces the ability of nerves to send signals. This leads to a variety of mental health and neurological problems.

Other Vitamins and Minerals

Many other vitamins and minerals are needed for mental well-being. They are needed to create neurotransmitters, regulate levels of neurotransmitters or hormones, and keep neurons working. These include other B vitamins such as B6 and B9 (folate), vitamin C, vitamin D, zinc, selenium, iodine, chromium, and electrolytes (sodium, potassium, calcium, and magnesium).

It would be overkill to initially test all of these purely for mental health reasons. Iron and B12 deficiencies are far more common causes of mental health symptoms. Many deficiencies are rare, especially with the number of foods being fortified with essential nutrients. After you've tried several treatments without success, testing for less common deficiencies may be warranted. You may have done the basic tests, tried a few medications, verified your diagnosis, and ruled out causes that won't respond to medications. That's the time to start considering more obscure causes.

Cost is also a factor. Consider vitamin D. Research in the early 2000s linked low vitamin D with various physical and mental illnesses. As a result, testing rates spiked at least 5–10 times in a few years. Testing among US Medicare beneficiaries increased 83 times. That cost adds up quickly.

Your body makes vitamin D when your skin is exposed to direct sunlight. Most people in northern countries such as Canada, where the sun is at a low angle much of the year, are probably deficient. However, five years' worth of a generic vitamin D supplement can cost less than a single test. It makes more financial sense to have everyone take a supplement and not test. Testing is therefore often not covered by insurance.

Still, many people are hesitant to take a supplement based on the assumption they're probably deficient. Showing them their actual vitamin D level may be enough to convince them to take it.

Hormones

Hormones are chemical messengers that regulate and control a wide range of body systems, including your mood. Your thyroid hormones are frequently checked by doctors when investigating mental health symptoms. The thyroid is a gland in your neck that makes hormones to regulate metabolism. An underactive thyroid can leave you fatigued, moody, or depressed. An overactive thyroid causes anxiety, irritability, and insomnia.

Blood tests can directly measure the thyroid hormones (T3 and T4). More often, a thyroid stimulating hormone (TSH) produced by the pituitary gland is measured instead. It's a more sensitive measure of thyroid problems. When you have symptoms of depression such as fatigue, your doctor is more likely to check your TSH than just prescribe an antidepressant.

While TSH is the only hormone routinely checked for mental health purposes, others may be checked in certain special cases. These include various sex hormones, including testosterone, estrogen, progesterone, and prolactin, as well as stress hormones including adrenaline, cortisol, and DHEA. And, of course, all these various hormones and neurotransmitters interact with one another. A problem with one is likely to cause ripple effects.

Other Blood Tests

Before prescribing any medications, your doctor may want to check your liver and kidneys, depending on your overall health.

Your liver metabolizes most medications, breaking them down into a form that can be directly used or into waste materials that can be removed. If your liver isn't working well, many medications won't work. Liver function tests (LFTs) measure levels of certain enzymes, e.g., ALT and AST.

Your kidneys filter out waste materials including many medications. If not working well, medications may build up to toxic levels. The most common test measures creatinine, a waste product from your muscles. Too much creatinine is a sign your kidneys aren't removing it well.

Other tests may help decide whether to use certain medications. As an example, some medications are more likely than others to increase cholesterol or blood glucose when taken for a long time. If your levels are already high, your doctor may want to monitor them more often if you do take the medication or decide to use a different medication altogether.

Some of your symptoms, mental health or otherwise, may cause your doctor to consider the possibility of another physical illness. If so, they may order other tests specifically for that condition.

Other Types of Tests

Beyond common blood tests, your doctor may order other tests.

The most routine is an electrocardiogram (ECG or EKG). This is a tracing of your heart's electrical activity recorded by multiple leads attached to your body. ECGs detect many structural or functional abnormalities in your heart such as a previous heart attack. Like testing cholesterol or glucose, an ECG helps your doctor decide how safe it is to use certain medications.

Certain older medications can worsen some heart problems. Alone or in combination, they can raise or lower your blood pressure, heart rate, or other measures that could magnify a borderline heart condition. A baseline ECG before you start a medication, or a check afterwards is a simple precaution that can prevent a very rare but serious outcome.[2]

One such measure is your *QT interval*, which is the length of time between two specific points in your heart rhythm. If it is much longer than normal, called *QT prolongation*, it puts you at risk of potentially dangerous heart rhythms. Many medications, including psychotropic medications (but also many antibiotics, antihistamines, gastrointestinal medications, cancer medications, and others) can increase the QT interval. It's rarely a problem unless it starts out very high (it can be inherited) or you take several medications that increase it. Tell your doctor about all your medications and supplements. Mention any heart problems you or any close relatives have.

Some symptoms may prompt your doctor to request a picture of your brain to look for any physical problems. This is not only to look for brain tumours but also various structural issues. Standard tests include a computed tomography (CT) or magnetic resonance imaging (MRI) scan. If something is out of whack with your hormones, they may even order scans for other parts of your body, such as your adrenal glands, which sit atop your kidneys.

While both CT and MRI scans of the brain are useful, each has advantages and disadvantages. CT, which use X-rays, may be faster or cheaper. CT is often the only option for very heavy patients or those who are claustrophobic. While MRI cannot be used safely if you have implanted metal of some kind, CT can be used. Either one can detect a wide range of problems, including bleeding and tumours, and both produce detailed images. MRI uses magnets and radio waves, so there is no concern of radiation exposure. MRI can more easily visualize some areas, such as the back of the brain, that CT cannot. MRI can pick up many differences in soft tissues, such as changes in the brain's white matter, that aren't visible with CT. The choice of which test to use will depend on what your doctor is looking for.

Newer imaging techniques include PET and SPECT scans. They show how different areas of the brain function, displaying higher or lower activity. Characteristic changes have been seen for several mental illnesses. While used mostly in larger centres now, expect their use to grow in future.

Another test is an electroencephalogram (EEG), which checks the electrical activity in the brain. Like an ECG, electrical leads are attached, this time to your head, and your brain waves are recorded. It's not a common test for mental health purposes. However, a few mental health symptoms, e.g., smelling things that aren't there, can be caused by certain seizure disorders, which an EEG can pick up.

Summary

- Lab investigations can detect many problems that contribute to mental health symptoms. Some vitamins and minerals are needed, directly or indirectly, to create neurotransmitters or help with their transmission.

- Iron deficiency is a very common cause of symptoms such as poor energy, concentration, and memory. There are many different ways to measure iron but, for mental health, serum ferritin should be evaluated. You will also need amounts higher than the normal ranges indicated on lab reports.

- Vitamin B12 deficiency also affects mental health symptoms. Other common tests include those for your thyroid (TSH), liver, and kidneys.

- An electrocardiogram (heart tracing) can check for rare but serious problems. Other tests can include imaging the structure of your brain (CT or MRI), its electrical activity (EEG), or its metabolism (PET or SPECT).

20

Lifestyle Factors

Because your physical and mental health are intertwined, the standard advice to improve your physical health—eat well, exercise, get plenty of sleep, don't drink too much alcohol—also applies to your mental health.

We'll look at several lifestyle factors here. Changes can both decrease the risk of developing new mental health symptoms and reduce the severity of existing ones. Many people try changing their diet, exercising, or limiting their alcohol use before trying other strategies to deal with their mental health problems. Such lifestyle changes may be all you need to treat mild symptoms. Even if they're not enough by themselves, lifestyle changes can reduce the time, dose, or effort you put into other treatments.

Negative lifestyle factors can worsen mental illness. They may become unhealthy means of coping, including comfort eating, smoking to relieve stress, or drinking alcohol in excess to forget problems.

Optimizing your physical health is a good idea at any time. Though difficult, most people at least know what's needed to improve their diet, increase exercise, or quit smoking. These changes can also be cost-effective. Few other mental health treatments are both as familiar and affordable.

Diet

There are some obvious links between diet and your mental health. From a psychological perspective, many people tie their body weight to their self-worth, a factor in depression. Taken further, eating disorders such as anorexia and bulimia are onerous mental illnesses. A fixation on body image can result in dangerous dietary changes. At a physical level, you can notice the effect that food has on your mood. You've likely experienced feeling happy and energetic after a light, nutrient-packed meal or sluggish and maybe even depressed after a large heavy meal. Food can literally affect your brain. There is a reason why you may crave chocolate. Chocolate can improve your mood or cognition because it ultimately increases serotonin.

A well-balanced diet consists of a broad range of whole foods along with good hydration. It contains many vitamins, minerals, proteins, carbohydrates, fats, and more. These provide your body with all the necessary building blocks it needs. As you've read, this includes your nervous system. It relies on multiple nutrients to assemble neurotransmitters and the right level of elements such as sodium and calcium to keep them moving.[1]

If you are severely deficient of a critical nutrient or can't absorb it, nothing but correcting the deficiency will fix the resulting problems. However, as you've read, tests for many deficiencies are not available or practical. Deficiencies in some nutrients have physical signs that your doctor or a naturopath may recognize. Trial and error with diet changes or supplements is sometimes the only way to know for sure.

Again, deficiencies to consider are iron, all B vitamins (especially B12), vitamin C, vitamin D, electrolytes, certain minerals (zinc, selenium, iodine, and chromium), and Omega-3 fatty acids. We'll discuss supplements in the next chapter.

But food is more than a collection of nutrients. Peoples' bodies have evolved to rely on whole foods in a variety of ways, such as helping with waste removal. Your digestive system processes whole foods at a pace that absorbs nutrients gradually. Too much simple sugar at once causes a spike in levels of the hormone insulin. That affects the brain and results in swings in energy and mood. Insulin production also frees up tryptophan which can be converted into serotonin. Very limited fad diets that focus on one ingredient, nutrient, or food group disrupt the body's normal functioning and can have their own effects on mood.

A well-balanced, nutrient-rich diet is an excellent way to protect or improve your mental health. If you need help with your diet, you can start by speaking with your doctor or a dietician. There are also many high quality books available.[2]

A properly functioning digestive system is needed to absorb nutrients for use elsewhere. Illnesses in your digestive tract can interfere with absorption. Changes in diet and health can affect your gut bacteria, which break down food into usable nutrients. That changes how well different nutrients are absorbed. For example, gut changes as people age lead to more problems absorbing vitamin B12. Different parts of the digestive tract absorb different nutrients, so surgeries removing parts of the digestive system can affect this.

Some illnesses lead to inflammation of the digestive system and elsewhere. Flare-ups of diseases such as Crohn's or ulcerative colitis often cause brain fog. This also happens to those with celiac disease who ingest gluten. These illnesses often start with vague symptoms. It can take years before they are diagnosed. The effect these have on absorption may not be the only factor. Researchers are also investigating how inflammation may affect mental health directly. The recent rise in food sensitivities and intolerances likely has mental health consequences.

Exercise

Like diet, exercise can reduce the incidence and severity of many physical illnesses. That, in turn, affects mental health. However, exercise can also directly affect mental health, especially depression. It both prevents symptoms from emerging and treats them when present.

On the prevention side, several recent large studies and systematic reviews are encouraging. As little as one hour of physical activity per week can reduce the risk of developing mild to moderate depression. Physical activity means not only exercise like running or lifting weights at the gym. Activities such as gardening, vacuuming, and dusting count, as long as your heart rate rises to a moderate level. People who are active, even if they are not fit, are at less risk for depression than fit people who are not active.

On the treatment side, studies show that exercise can be as effective as an antidepressant for mild to moderate depression. Exercise further combats depressive symptoms when added to an antidepressant. The results are pretty good for anxiety, too. There, exercise has been found as effective as cognitive behavioural therapy.

Exercise and physical activity improve serotonin levels. They release endorphins (neurotransmitters having an opioid-like effect) and cannabinoids (which enhance some neural receptors). They also lower the stress hormone cortisol. Exercise and physical activity also strengthen a part of the brain that helps with memory and emotion.

Recommendations for the type and amount of exercise vary. Both cardiovascular and resistance exercise have shown clear mental health benefits. A good target is 30 minutes of moderate intensity exercise per day, but even small amounts of physical activity help. This is good news, particularly if you've not been very active. Start small and increase at a pace that works for you. Your doctor can help with any concerns about increasing your activity.

Interestingly, there is mixed evidence about high-intensity exercise for mental health. Some studies support it while others are more cautious. High-intensity exercise does increase cortisol levels, albeit briefly. Injuries from high-intensity exercise can cause longer-term cortisol increases. Prolonged high cortisol leaves you activated, in a low-grade fight-or-flight mode, which creates many adverse effects, including anxiety.

Finally, some recent work has shown that time spent outdoors in a natural environment benefits mental health. Countless walkers, hikers, runners, and cyclists find that the combination of physical activity in the great outdoors is hard to beat.

Sleep

Like poor diet and lack of exercise, poor sleep is implicated in multiple physical and mental health problems. Insomnia (difficulty falling or staying asleep) is a symptom of several mental illnesses. Many sleep disorders are considered forms of mental illness in their own right. Addressing sleep problems reduces the risk of developing some mental illnesses and can treat existing ones. Poor sleep and illnesses such as depression or anxiety create a mutually reinforcing feedback loop.

Poor sleep, even for a short while, can lead to increased irritability, anger, stress, and depression. It also affects short- and long-term memory, attention, planning, and motivation. Extreme sleep deprivation can lead to paranoia and hallucinations. For those with a bipolar disorder, poor sleep increases the risk of developing hypomania or mania.

If you have difficulty falling asleep or staying asleep, aren't rested upon waking, or if you are tired during the day, poor sleep is likely an issue. Do you snore, sometimes wake up choking or gasping, or has your partner noticed you sometimes stop breathing for a few seconds? You may suffer from sleep apnea, reducing oxygen to your brain and body. That can lead to memory problems, trouble concentrating, and mood swings. An overnight sleep study at a dedicated sleep lab can tell you a lot about your sleep. You can also borrow equipment to test for sleep apnea at home.

Depending on the exact problem, there are many effective treatments available. The first option is usually improving your *sleep hygiene,* a term for various behavioural and environmental factors. These include avoiding naps or caffeine late in the day, keeping a consistent schedule, developing sleep rituals, not consuming media in bed, and so on. Other treatments may include mechanical devices, cognitive behavioural therapy, and for occasional use, some herbal, over-the-counter, or prescription medications.[3]

If you suspect poor sleep may be a factor in your mental (or physical) health, speak with your doctor.

Caffeine

Caffeine is highly addictive, yet legal and virtually unregulated. It's the most widely consumed psychoactive drug in the world, regularly used by more than 80% of adults. We're both happy to be included in this group.

Not to put too fine a point on it, excessive caffeine is anxiety in a cup (or can, pill, candy, or gourd). It causes jitteriness, restlessness, palpitations, nausea, dizziness, and insomnia. These are indistinguishable from symptoms you'd experience during a panic attack. Caffeine increases adrenaline and cortisol, decreases the calming neurotransmitter GABA, increases blood pressure, and decreases blood flow to the brain. Yet, modest amounts of caffeine can reduce fatigue and tiredness. It can improve concentration, coordination, and athletic performance. It even reduces the risk of depression or suicide by about 15-20%.

What is a modest amount depends on your weight and tolerance. On average, an 8 ounce cup of brewed coffee contains about 100 mg of caffeine but may have up to double that. Typical cup sizes in most North American coffee shops range from 50–150% larger than that. This can put one drink at close to 500 mg of caffeine. Both Health Canada and the FDA suggest a maximum of 400 mg per day is safe for average adults. Most people will experience the effects of caffeine at less than a quarter of that amount.

Caffeine is often combined with other stimulants such as tobacco or sugar in energy drinks and many popular beverages at chain coffee shops. Mixing caffeine and alcohol (a depressant) can mask the body's normal reaction to consuming too much alcohol, leading to significant intoxication. Caffeine can also interact with many medications.

If you suffer from significant anxiety, reducing your caffeine intake will likely help. Large decreases can have profound effects. Like any drug that creates physical dependence, decrease slowly and gradually. Withdrawal symptoms include headaches, irritability, poor concentration, and fatigue.

Start by accurately determining your caffeine intake. Then discuss with your doctor if reducing it might help your symptoms.

Tobacco

Tobacco contains the addictive stimulant nicotine. It has some of the same benefits as caffeine, particularly improving concentration. However, it can also play havoc with your mental health. Biologically, nicotine affects the transmission of the excitatory neurotransmitters glutamate and acetylcholine. This, in turn, releases norepinephrine, epinephrine, serotonin, and dopamine. All of this leads to the pleasure that smokers and other nicotine users crave. Unfortunately, the effect doesn't last. Nicotine is associated with an increased risk of developing depression long term.

Many people smoke as a coping mechanism during times of stress. Yet, tobacco users have higher levels of stress and anxiety. This grows with time and as tolerance increases. Short-term improvements ("I need a cigarette to relax") are fleeting. They don't offset the elevated anxiety levels caused by nicotine use. Nicotine interacts with many medications including some used in mental health. If your smoking habits change, ask your doctor if this could affect the dose of your medications. Even in small amounts, the long-term risks to your mental and physical health outweigh any benefits.

Alcohol

Alcohol is primarily a depressant, though it also has some stimulant effects on neurotransmitters. That makes for a careful balance between enjoyment and discomfort that can easily swing from one to the other. Experiences vary. Alcohol tends to decrease the activity of neurotransmitters, including glutamate, and binds to GABA receptors, increasing transmission. This results in relaxation, but also impaired balance and memory. It raises the activity of other neurotransmitters, including dopamine (pleasure) and norepinephrine (energy and motivation). It also raises serotonin, but unfortunately, the serotonin receptor affected increases nausea.

Alcohol temporarily reduces anxiety. It provides the "liquid courage" that helps you overcome social anxiety. Afterwards, however, anxiety is increased, and alcohol metabolites increase anxiety levels and remain in the brain for several days. Anxiety worsens as dependence increases. Alcohol can bring on temporary but severe depressive symptoms. Longer-term use starts looking like a depressive disorder. In some people, these symptoms will resolve after several weeks without drinking. In people with a bipolar disorder, however, alcohol can be enough to trigger mood episodes.

Consuming alcohol amounts to consuming low nutrient liquid calories. It either replaces healthy food or adds unneeded calories to your diet. Diets associated with alcohol use increase the risk of protein and energy deficiencies. They also lead to decreases in multiple B vitamins, as well as elements such as magnesium and zinc. These affect mood. Alcohol decreases the absorption and storage of thiamine (vitamin B1). Severe thiamine deficiency can lead to permanent brain damage and even death.

Like caffeine and nicotine, alcohol can produce physical dependence. This leads to intense withdrawal symptoms including seizures if abruptly discontinued. The family and societal costs of excess alcohol are devastating and well known. If alcohol is an issue for you, your doctor or a local support line can discuss resources in your area.

Cannabis

Using cannabis for mental health purposes is both widely promoted and criticized. Some claim it is a cure for every physical and mental problem under the sun. Others are equally quick to proclaim the incredible danger and condemn it out of hand.

What do we know? Not as much as we should. First, legal availability is rapidly shifting and varies by jurisdiction. It ranges from outright prohibition to legalized recreational use with minimal restrictions. In between are a range of restrictions on medicinal usage, types of products, distribution channels, and so on. Policy decisions are often based on politics more than evidence. The legal framework has made it extremely difficult for health researchers. That leaves a lack of high-quality, rigorous data. Solid evidence supports use only for chronic pain, some types of seizures, and nausea from chemotherapy. These legal issues and limited evidence affect health professionals including doctors. Most regulatory bodies now err on the side of caution. Except in specific cases, they recommend doctors not endorse cannabis use with their patients.

Despite all this, cannabis is readily available. It is widely used both medicinally and recreationally across a broad demographic range. Here in BC, the province has long embraced cannabis use. It's known as the best quality producer in North America (we've been told). Usage rates are the highest in Canada at 17.3%. Total cannabis use in Canada is on par with tobacco.[4] Some consumers are incredibly well informed about the effects of different cannabis strains and products. Most consumers, however, have little appreciation of this. Potential users need more education.

The active agents in cannabis plants are chemicals called *cannabinoids*. There are over 100 different varieties. Our body naturally produces similar

> chemicals called *endocannabinoids*. Both act as neurotransmitters that affect the endocannabinoid system, which controls many bodily and neural functions. The best-known cannabinoids are tetrahydrocannabinol (THC), the primary intoxicating component of cannabis plants, and cannabidiol (CBD), which is not intoxicating. Different species of plants, or strains, contain different amounts of each cannabinoid. This results in often markedly different effects for different strains. Each person also responds to these chemicals differently. Finally, strains are categorized as either *indica, sativa,* or hybrids of the two. These two main species of cannabis have broadly different physical characteristics. However, these categories tell you very little about the cannabinoid content or even effects of individual strains.

Potential Risks

To date, most studies of cannabis use and mental health have not distinguished among different strains. Yet, the majority of recreational strains are bred with ever-increasing amounts of the intoxicating cannabinoid THC. This makes for a more potent high (hence, "this isn't the same weed your parents were smoking in the 60's"). THC can cause anxiety, psychosis, and mood symptoms in some users. However, much of the cannabis for medical use has less THC and more of the non-intoxicating cannabinoid CBD. Medical use has been a small segment of the market until recently. We can infer that most cannabis in past studies had high levels of THC.

There are two main concerns about cannabis use. The first is impairment. Cannabis can affect tasks, such as driving, just as alcohol does. The second is its effect on young people, whose minds are still developing (typically, until age 25). Many studies correlate early cannabis use with schizophrenia and an earlier onset of psychosis. This suggests caution is warranted, particularly in those with existing psychosis or where genetic risk is present.

Increased risk has also been suggested for those with bipolar disorder or a genetic predisposition toward it. This includes having close relatives with either depression or a bipolar disorder. These people may have an earlier onset of bipolar disorder, longer or more severe periods of hypomania or mania, and increased risk of suicide attempts.

The depth and breadth of the data supporting these risks is limited and suspect. At the same time, there is no hard data to show that cannabis use reduces the risk of mental health issues.

Continued use despite clinical impairment is considered a cannabis use disorder. It's associated with more negative outcomes across a range of mental health disorders. Some studies show a modestly larger risk of depression for light users (17% higher), greater with heavy users (to 62% higher). Studies also show higher risks of anxiety disorders, and anxiety is common with (primarily THC-dominant) cannabis. Neurocognitive deficits (e.g., memory, attention) among heavy users are widely seen, during and shortly after use. Nothing conclusively suggests these effects are permanent, especially for those over 25 years old.

Cannabis, like many substances, interacts with many different prescription medications. This includes antidepressants or other psychotropic medications. It may increase or decrease side effects or even the effectiveness of medications. The dosage of some medications is fairly fussy so that a change in cannabis use may be enough to throw things off. If you are using cannabis, let prescribers know that, along with any changes to your usage.

Potential Benefits

Much of the interest in cannabis for mental health is directed toward CBD-dominant strains or their extracts. Most recreational cannabis, with more THC and other intoxicating cannabinoids, is likely less helpful.

CBD has been widely thought to improve multiple forms of anxiety. This is an area of active behavioural and biological research. CBD has anecdotal evidence for treating depression. Some tentative information points to the use of CBD as an antipsychotic. Other possible effects on brain health are at the early stage of research, and specific mechanisms are unclear. Research in animal models suggests that CBD may affect serotonin transmission.

The lack of rigorous data makes it impractical to draw any definitive conclusions on the mental health benefits of CBD. The relaxing legal climate will lead to more rigorous evaluation in future, both for treating existing conditions and examining its effect on developing mental illness.

One exception to the focus on CBD is for those with insomnia or nightmares. Many find that higher THC strains help with these symptoms. It's widely used by military veterans with PTSD, who also find it decreases hyperarousal symptoms. Chronic pain is also very common in this group. A variety of strains, some THC-dominant, are reportedly effective here.

> We're still in the "Wild West" stage of cannabis use for mental health. For those who choose to use cannabis, a risk reduction model is advised. The Lower-Risk Cannabis Use Guidelines (LRCUG) available through the Centre for Addiction and Mental Health (CAMH) are a good starting point.[5]

Illicit Drugs

This topic could fill a book on its own. However, we won't have a lot to say in this book about illicit drugs and mental health. Many of them have a high potential for addiction. There are often negative effects when coming down from a high. Immediate and longer-term safety concerns are also a factor.

Not surprisingly, most of them work on neurotransmitters. Cocaine, methamphetamine, and many others work on dopamine. Cocaine, LSD, and ecstasy work on serotonin. Cocaine and methamphetamine work on norepinephrine. Ketamine works on glutamate. Many illicit drugs are chemically similar to other neurotransmitters and bind to their receptors (e.g., opioids, psilocybin).

Interestingly, academic researchers are investigating using various illicit or heavily regulated drugs (e.g., ketamine, GHB, MDMA) as well as hallucinogens (e.g., LSD, psilocybin) to treat depression.[6] But, these are still early days.

Summary

- Lifestyle changes can reduce the chance of developing mental illness and can treat many milder cases of mental illness. These changes are a very common first approach to dealing with mental health problems.

- A well-balanced, nutrient-rich whole food diet is the best way for most people to obtain all the necessary building blocks for good mental health.

- Even small amounts of exercise can have mental health benefits. Regular exercise may be as effective as an antidepressant for mild depression and anxiety or reduce the necessary antidepressant dose.

- Poor sleep can cause serious mental health problems in a short period. Medications or supplements can help for occasional problems, while better sleep hygiene, therapy, or other treatments can be used long term.

- Caffeine, tobacco, alcohol, cannabis, and illicit drugs can all play havoc with your mental health. If you have anxiety, seriously consider your caffeine intake.

21

Vitamins and Supplements

Some people choose to take vitamins, herbs, and other natural supplements to help with their physical or mental health, or both. *Complementary and Alternative Medicine* (CAM) is the blanket term covering these, along with treatments such as acupuncture and massage. Some people rely solely on CAM treatments, avoiding treatments such as pharmaceuticals recommended by medical doctors. Most CAM users, however, combine the two.

While usage varies by country and culture, CAM practices are widespread. One American survey examined people self-identifying as having "anxiety attacks" or "severe depression."[1] Approximately 55% used one or more CAM therapies as part of their treatment. Around 20% of survey respondents saw a CAM provider while about 66% saw a conventional provider (e.g., doctor, psychologist, social worker, or clergy). There was likely some overlap between the two.

A broader American survey reported on CAM usage for all illnesses, not only mental health.[2] It identified anxiety and depression as two of the most frequent conditions for which people rely on CAM. These were below only back and neck problems (people seeking mostly chiropractic care and massage treatments).

Can supplements cure mental illness? It depends. As you have learned, mental illness varies greatly between people, and is caused by many factors. Symptoms and severity may differ. Be wary of any treatment promoted as a universal cure for even a single mental illness.

We'll loosely divide the various supplements into three categories: those that address nutritional deficiencies, those related to neurotransmitters and hormones, and plants and herbs whose extracts are used medicinally.

Nutritional Deficiencies

We'll start with supplements that address nutritional deficiencies. As you know, many nutrients are needed for the proper functioning of the nervous system. If you aren't deficient in a nutrient, is taking a supplement helpful? Are there benefits to boosting your level much higher than normal? In general, the answer is a clear no. Your body uses only what it needs. At best, excess intake of supplements will result in very expensive urine. At worst, high levels of some nutrients can be toxic. Furthermore, your body maintains a delicate equilibrium between certain combinations of nutrients. A large excess of one can quickly turn into a deficiency of another.

How much of each nutrient do you need, from food or supplements? National standards for dietary intake provide the most reliable recommendations.[3] While you may need more or less for particular health reasons, any large deviations should occur under medical supervision.

Even with an iffy diet, many people only require a well-rounded multivitamin. Additional iron, vitamin B12, vitamin C, and vitamin D supplementation may be needed by some. Be wary of vitamin, mineral, or other micronutrient blends said to benefit mental health. If you decide to use supplements, let your choice be guided by specific deficiencies found in your laboratory testing. Read the labels. Keep in mind the maximum healthy intake of each nutrient. More is not better.

Neurotransmitters and Hormones

The second category of supplements are those related to neurotransmitters or hormones, including their building blocks.

You saw that a shortage of neurotransmitters can lead to mental health symptoms. You need raw materials, known as precursors, to create them. If you don't have enough raw materials, you won't have enough neurotransmitters. Supplements are one way to obtain those precursors.

> Why not take a supplement made of a neurotransmitter itself? Why take precursors? Wouldn't skipping the middleman be more efficient?
> Unfortunately, ingested neurotransmitters can't reach the brain where they are needed. This is because of the *blood-brain barrier* (BBB). The BBB is a membrane that separates blood vessels from the brain. It permits only some molecules to cross from the bloodstream into the brain. Very small

> molecules can cross. An elaborate system of transporters helps certain other molecules cross. Molecules without a transporter can't cross.
>
> For example, serotonin does not cross the BBB, but 5-HTP, a serotonin precursor, does. Once in the brain, it can then be processed (with help from other vitamins and minerals) into serotonin. That's why there are 5-HTP supplements, but not ones containing serotonin itself.

Like vitamins and minerals, precursor supplements address existing deficiencies, but won't help if you're not deficient. Other approaches, such as changing your diet, can do the same thing. Taking more than you need won't help more. Remember, too, that vitamins and minerals, which make up precursors, are used for more than building neurotransmitters. Supplementing only with precursors may neglect these other roles.

Tryptophan and 5-HTP

Tryptophan is an essential amino acid. Your body needs it to function, but can't make it from other chemicals. It's widely found in our diet, especially in protein-rich foods. Your body converts tryptophan into a precursor called 5-HTP, which is then converted into serotonin. Tryptophan or 5-HTP supplements may provide a small improvement in depressive symptoms for some. Presumably, these people are deficient. However, such supplements have not been proven to be the safe, side-effect free, and effective natural replacements for serotonergic antidepressants that many had hoped.[4]

S-adenosylmethionine (SAMe)

SAMe is naturally found in your body. It helps create and destroy neurotransmitters. The liver makes SAMe from vitamins B6, B9 (folic acid), B12, and an essential amino acid called methionine. As B9 and B12 deficiencies are common, a deficiency of SAMe would not be unusual. In those cases, SAMe supplements can improve mild depressive symptoms or boost the effects of antidepressants in those who had a limited response.[5] If you have a bipolar disorder, be aware that SAMe can trigger hypomania or mania.

GABA

GABA is the main inhibitory neurotransmitter in your body. Many medications for anxiety increase GABA transport in the nervous system. This slows other signals and improves anxiety and insomnia. Just as it does with other neurotransmitters, your body creates GABA. Like serotonin, GABA can't reach the brain, so GABA supplements aren't effective. The medications gabapentin and pregabalin, used for pain, seizures, and anxiety, are almost identical to GABA, but different enough that they can reach the brain.

Omega-3 Fatty Acids

One trendy supplement is Omega-3 (found in fish, flax, etc.). It has been widely investigated for use in unipolar and bipolar depression, ADHD, and aggression and impulsivity in borderline personality disorder.[6] The eicosapentaenoic acid (EPA) form of Omega-3 appears to have a greater effect on depressive symptoms than the docosahexaenoic acid (DHA) form. It has a good safety profile and reported benefits in other areas. It seems likely that a deficiency could modestly worsen some mental health symptoms.

Melatonin

This natural hormone regulates body rhythms, synchronizing them with day and night. It's widely used as a short-term or long-term sleep aid. It also relieves jet lag. Many studies show positive effects, though there are concerns over the quality of the studies themselves.[7]

L-Theanine

This chemical, found in high amounts in green tea, has long been used for relaxation.[8] Good evidence supports this effect. It inhibits the excitatory neurotransmitter glutamate, as well as increasing GABA. Combined with caffeine (as found naturally in tea), it increases attention, improves cognition, and reduces the jitters when compared to intake of caffeine alone. No clear evidence, however, supports its use to treat clinical anxiety disorders.

Inositol

Inositol aids neurotransmitter activity within neurons. It is found in a variety of foods, and the body can create it from glucose. A few small studies suggest inositol supplements may somewhat help depression, bipolar depression, panic, and OCD.[9] Inositol is also sold, usually with choline, as a cognition and memory enhancer. Evidence that inositol supplements can affect mental health is limited and primarily anecdotal.

Choline

Choline plays many roles in the body. It's a building block for the neurotransmitter acetylcholine, which is critical for memory formation and prenatal brain development. The body makes some, but not enough. The best sources are liver, eggs, and peanuts, the food additive lecithin, along with various meat, fish, and dairy sources. Some studies show choline supplements improve cognitive performance.[10] Many medications have anticholinergic properties that negatively affect memory and cognition and cause other physical side effects. Choline supplements may help with these problems.

Phenylalanine and Tyrosine

Phenylalanine is an essential amino acid found in many protein-rich foods. It is converted into tyrosine, which is then converted into the neurotransmitters dopamine and norepinephrine. A shortage of phenylalanine or tyrosine decreases dopamine and norepinephrine just as a shortage of tryptophan decreases serotonin. Taking phenylalanine or tyrosine may help with cognition in healthy people under short-term stress. Acute stress causes a rapid turnover of neurotransmitters and therefore potential deficits.[11]

Herbals

The final category of supplements we'll cover are plants, herbs, and their extracts. Plants have been used medicinally for thousands of years for mental health. Given the desire of many people to pursue natural treatments instead of manufactured pharmaceuticals, they continue to be used extensively. Or as the introduction to one fairly typical article[12] puts it:

> Want to relieve your depression symptoms using safe, natural antidepressants? Want an herbal alternative that can improve your depression symptoms without antidepressant side effects?

Do herbals deliver on this promise? Applying modern standards of evidence to herbal treatments has been challenging.[13] Only two herbal supplements have been rigorously studied (including reviews and meta-analyses) and found to help in specific situations.

St. John's Wort

St. John's wort[14] is probably the single most used herbal remedy in mental health. It has been studied extensively and found to be more effective than placebo at treating mild to moderate depression. A few studies found it has a comparable effect to some (older) antidepressants. It has not been shown, however, to help with other mental illnesses, including any form of anxiety.

It has a multitude of effects on several neurotransmitters, most notably serotonin. Unfortunately, it seriously interacts with many herbal and prescription medications, including migraine medications, birth control pills, heart medications, cancer medications, HIV/AIDS medications, pain medications, blood thinners, and most psychotropic medications. In combination with other medications, it can lead to serotonin syndrome (we'll discuss this in the chapter titled *Antidepressants*). If you take St. John's wort, it's critical to make sure your doctors and pharmacist know.

Kava

St. John's wort can help with depression but not anxiety. One plant studied extensively for anxiety is kava,[15] native to the western Pacific islands. It can modestly improve generalized anxiety disorder when used up to 24 weeks.

Safety concerns regarding liver damage (sometimes fatal) and medication interactions have dogged kava. For years, it was banned outright in some countries, including the UK, Canada, and EU member states. Further investigations have shown that peeled kava root extracted with water (how it was traditionally used) is safe. Virtually all bans have been since replaced by strict regulations on sales and imports. Use caution. Take kava supplements from a regulated source. Be very careful with alcohol or medications that are metabolized by the liver. If you have liver problems, don't take kava.

Other

Many other herbals are promoted for their mental health benefits. The evidence supporting them is much weaker than for St. John's wort or kava. We list the main ones in Table 21.1. The evidence column grades the current state of evidence, as determined by a large review of herbals.[16] Even the best (A) have very little evidence compared to St. John's wort or kava. No herbals have close to the amount of evidence as psychotropic medications or have been shown to help with anything but mild mental illness.

General Cautions

The decision about whether to try a particular natural supplement is not an easy one. Here, we touch on a few factors to consider.

Limited Studies

As we've seen, there is a lack of high-quality scientific evidence about the safety and efficacy of many herbal treatments. There are limitations in the

Table 21.1: Other herbal supplements.

Herbal medicine	Condition	Evidence
Ashwagandha *(Withania somnifera)*	Anxiety	C
Borage *(Echium amoenum)*	Depression	B
	OCD	B
Chamomile *(Matricaria recutita)*	Anxiety	B
Ginkgo *(Ginkgo biloba)*	Anxiety	B
Lavender *(Lavandula spp.)*	Depression	B-
Lemon balm *(Melissa officinalis)*	Anxiety	C
Passionflower *(Passiflora incarnata)*	Anxiety	B
	Insomnia	C
Roseroot *(Rhodiola rosea)*	Depression	B
Saffron *(Crocus sativus)*	Depression	A
Skullcap *(Scutellaria lateriflora)*	Anxiety	C
Turmeric *(Curcuma longa)*	Depression	C
Valerian *(Valeriana spp.)*	Insomnia	C

size of studies, methodology, measurement, study participants, controls, and many other areas.

Standards

You can grow St. John's wort in your backyard garden. However, most people using medicinal plants use commercially produced supplements. While prescription medications are closely regulated in most countries, herbal supplements are not as strictly regulated. That puts a much greater onus on you to ensure you're getting what you think you are.

In Canada, these are termed *natural health products*. They must be registered with Health Canada, who assign an NPN (Natural Product Number). Information must be supplied regarding all ingredients, source, dose, and recommended use. Little evidence is required showing the product is useful though. Safety is judged solely on the acceptability and quantity of each ingredient. In the USA, these are referred to as *dietary supplements*. They aren't registered with the FDA, but ingredient information such as quantity and source must be provided on the product label.

> Notably, independent confirmation of safety, efficacy for any given purpose, and consistent quantities and strengths of ingredients are not required for these products. Even in the case of well-known brands, there can be wide variations for some substances. While most established manufacturers are presumably well-meaning, trustworthy and conscientious, the lax regulations do make abuse of the system easy.[17]

Natural Medicine is Medicine

Despite being a natural product, natural medicine is still medicine.

It can help your symptoms, have negative effects, cause reactions and illnesses, and even be toxic. It can interact with other medications, natural or pharmaceutical. Those interactions can be potentially dangerous. Many substances, natural or otherwise, affect the liver, where they are metabolized. This can lead to either a toxic build-up or drastic reduction of other medications in your system. Even something as innocuous as grapefruit juice can interact with many medications. Ensure your doctors or pharmacist know everything you take, including herbal products.[18]

Like other treatments, natural supplements need to work on the problem you're actually having. Most mental illnesses such as anxiety and depression have a multitude of possible causes. A treatment that works to address one cause (e.g., a deficiency) won't help if your illness is caused by something else.

Summary

- Vitamins, herbs, and other natural supplements are very commonly used treatments for a wide range of mental health conditions.
- To be effective, you must match the right supplement to the right underlying cause, e.g. a deficiency in a vitamin or other neurotransmitter precursor.
- Herbals and supplements are less regulated than pharmaceutical medications, and there's less money to research their effectiveness. Be skeptical of any products promoted as a universal cure.
- Like pharmaceuticals, natural products can interact with other medications or supplements. Tell your doctor or pharmacist about everything you take.

22

Talk Therapy

One of the best-known tools in mental health is talk therapy. It goes by various names: therapy, psychotherapy, counselling, analysis, and many more. As with so many aspects of mental health, you likely have an idea of what therapy entails. Yet, most people don't know how to tell the different forms apart, how to choose between them, how they work, or how they can help.

You may have already tried therapy and found it didn't help. Don't skip this chapter. There are hundreds of different therapies. Some therapies are more general and can help with a wider range of problems; others are useful only in specific situations. Is therapy right for you? It depends on your problem. Someone saying that therapy will solve your mental health problem—not knowing what it is—makes no sense.

There are many types of therapies, but far more therapists. Each uses a different set of therapies, putting their unique spin on each one. Success depends on the right therapy used in the right way for the right problem. Some problems won't respond to any therapy, while others are well suited to many forms of therapy.

In this chapter, we'll give you a very broad overview highlighting the diversity of therapy. You'll get a sense of what therapy can and can't do for your mental health. We'll also identify a few common types of therapies that have good clinical evidence to support them. More are described in *Appendix B*. In the process, you'll learn some of the questions to ask as you explore what might be right for you.

In the following chapter, we'll discuss how to find the right therapist. Therapy is less regulated and standardized than, for example, pharmaceutical treatments. Be warned that the "experts" you meet may not know what techniques would be helpful in your situation.

What Does Therapy Look Like?

Gone are the days where a Freud-like psychoanalyst pensively sits back in their chair while you lay on a long couch. Ditto for interpreting ink blots. Sure, you'll find these still used today but very rarely. Therapy today can take on all kinds of different forms:

- Therapy may be delivered one on one, therapist and patient. A therapist may also work with two people (not necessarily romantically linked), a few more people (such as a family), a small group, or even quite large groups.

- The therapist may be a trained mental health professional such as a psychiatrist, psychologist, clinical counsellor, or a psychiatric nurse. They may be a social worker or a religious leader. They may even be a peer in your workplace, a close family member, or an empathetic friend. In some therapeutic interactions, none of the participants has any mental health or therapy training at all. This is not uncommon in groups that follow a particular structure or set of rules. Others can be even more laissez-faire.

- Therapy may occur in an office, a living room, a classroom, a community centre, a library, a yoga studio, a hospital, or a mental health clinic. It may take place over the telephone with a worker at a crisis centre, during a Skype video chat with a faraway therapist, or while alone with a workbook or an iPhone app.

- Therapy may be a brief, one-time conversation, or a monthly two-hour meeting. It may be one hour a week for a couple of months, or several hours a few days a week, possibly for years. It can follow a consistent schedule and frequency or may vary with circumstances.

The Right Therapy For You

Counsellors, psychologists, and other providers employ many different therapy techniques. Some of these have been studied extensively and have good evidence behind them. Others have been the topic of fewer studies but are commonly used and effective. Still others may be more obscure, novel, or fringe; perhaps helpful for some people, perhaps not. In practice, most providers draw from several different techniques, choosing what they feel is appropriate given your situation. Relatively few are purists who strictly adhere to a single methodology.

As with all things mental health, there is no one-size-fits-all solution when it comes to therapy. If you're sick and someone tells you that, "You should take something for that," it leaves more questions than answers. Sick with what? What medicine? Prescription, over-the-counter, herbal? How will it help? Who should I get it from? Hearing "you should go talk to a therapist" should prompt similar questions. What problem needs fixing? What technique should be used? How will it help? Who should I talk to?

Any therapy you choose should help you achieve the goals described in your living treatment plan. You need to ask questions up front to see if it's right for you and track your progress during treatment (we'll discuss managing therapy shortly). All therapies presumably aim to make things better. You need to narrow down your choices to find the type of therapy that best fits your situation. This can be very difficult, especially on your own, so ask your doctor or others you trust for help.

There are as many ways to categorize types of therapy as there are people writing about them. We won't abandon that tradition here. We'll discuss four general approaches to therapy, with the goal of helping you pick which might fit your situation. The approaches are *practical advice, skills and techniques, depth,* and *eclectic.* Keep in mind these are our terms. There is always considerable overlap in any categorization.

Practical Advice

Practical advice helps you through situations you're facing right now.

When you're having difficulty with a situation at home, work, or elsewhere, a therapist can help you deal with the problem and move forward. Experiencing grief due to a death in the family? Struggling to cope financially after a job loss? Overwhelmed juggling too many responsibilities? Not sure how to respond to bullying at work? Don't know what to say to your teenager? Need help making a stressful decision about your relationship?

A therapist can help you identify the cause of your distress and what to do about it. They can help you find alternatives, pros and cons, and see things from different perspectives. They may even role-play situations with you to increase your confidence. Sometimes, talking things out with someone who is not directly involved is all you need.

Though highly trained professionals may be better at providing this support, they're not the only ones who do. Support can also come from volunteers at a mental health support telephone line or others with mental illness in a peer support group. It can come from friends and family.

Finding better ways to deal with your current situation may even help you in the future. But that isn't the goal. Therapy providing practical advice is all about working through struggles you're dealing with in the present.

Is what you're going through now a one-off situation? Focused practical advice might be just what you need. Do similar problems seem to keep cropping up for you again and again? Practical advice may get you through the current round. But, you'll need something more if you don't want to end up back at square one next time.

Skills and Techniques

The second general category of talk therapy teaches you skills and techniques. These help you gain control of overwhelming emotions and longstanding distorted thoughts. These worsen when you have a mental illness. You learn skills and techniques to apply to a current stressor. This helps in the short term. Over time and with practice, you confidently use the skills or techniques in various situations that you later face.

In these types of therapies, the therapist or provider acts as a teacher. Given individual situations are not the focus but only serve as examples used to apply the skill, these skills and techniques can be taught to several people at once. Groups can be offered relatively affordably and are often supported by governments or other organizations. In a group, you learn from others experiencing similar problems and realize you're not alone. Other categories of talk therapies are less suited to group delivery.

There are many different types of skills or techniques. A few prominent examples are described here:

- *Grounding Techniques.* When you are very overwhelmed or panicked, your brain flips into a basic fight-or-flight mode. Your heart beats faster, your breathing quickens, you feel pumped up and full of adrenaline. Other parts of your brain fade deep into the background, including those that control reasoning and problem solving. Grounding techniques are simple exercises that switch your brain out of fight-or-flight mode. This, in turn, reactivates your ability to problem solve and think through your situation.

- *Mindfulness.* Many people go through life on autopilot, jumping from one task to the next. You may be constantly distracted by things around you, other people, or notifications from your phone. Those things in themselves can increase stress. Mindfulness is a set of meditative practices that encourage you to be present and more aware of how you're feeling. Among other benefits, mindfulness helps you lower your baseline level of stress and anxiety. You'll likely deal with a stressful situation far better if you're relaxed to start with, instead of almost at the point of snapping. You'll be able to respond instead of just react. Scientific studies have shown multiple mental and physical health benefits of living mindfully.

- *Cognitive Behavioural Therapy (CBT).* One of the most-studied therapies, CBT in its various forms is a collection of skills that help you improve emotional reactions, and change thoughts and patterns of behaviour. It teaches you questions to ask yourself when placed in a difficult situation, and methods you can use to approach and break down problems. With continued practice, automatic but unhelpful thoughts, feelings, and behaviours are gradually replaced by more constructive ones. Extensive data, including from advanced brain imaging techniques, have shown that over the long term, CBT often results in improvement comparable to medications.

- *Dialectical Behavioural Therapy (DBT).* Intense emotion can lead to impulsive behaviour, self-harm, and substance use. DBT is a multi-faceted program to help those who frequently experience such emotion. It was initially designed to treat borderline personality disorder but has been used, in whole or in part, for many other disorders including depression, PTSD, binge eating, and addiction. DBT programs interweave aspects of all three of the previous skills and techniques, plus many others.

The skills themselves are general and can be applied to many situations. The trick is learning how to apply the skill or technique to new situations you encounter (and remembering to do so). As part of learning, you work through exercises or scenarios where you try to apply the technique. With practice, doing this becomes ingrained. However, learning the skill in session and then immediately forgetting it won't be of much help.

Depth

We're calling the third category of talk therapies depth therapies. They help you develop a better understanding of yourself, based on past events and experiences. You learn how your past has influenced your current thoughts and behaviours. With this new self-knowledge, you construct a new and healthier approach to future events and circumstances.

In depth therapies, a therapist helps you identify and process past events and themes that make up your current psyche. They then help you build up a new foundation. This is what most people initially think of when you mention therapy (couches, cigars, and similar clichés optional). Depth therapies are very much geared toward improving your future situation. Digging into your past usually leaves you feeling worse before you feel better.

Psychoanalysis, as exemplified by people such as Freud and Jung, started in the late 1800s. It has branched into many, many approaches and schools of thought. Today, there are huge variations, some of which have been well studied. Thankfully, many modern forms are also far less time-intensive. They are practiced almost exclusively one on one, are generally not amenable to groups, and do not aim to provide practical advice.

Eclectic

The final category of talk therapy is eclectic therapy. This category is a mix of the previous three categories. Therapists who don't focus exclusively on a particular type of therapy often practice some form of eclectic therapy. They mix techniques to meet your needs, and share some common characteristics:

- The tone of the therapy is generally positive. Therapists encourage you and help build your confidence. You achieve this through quick, identifiable progress with current problems and stressors.
- They take into account key events and broad themes from your past. They don't delve as far as depth therapies, so are less time-consuming. Therapists may use techniques such as short-term psychodynamic therapy to capture and frame themes. They help you gain insight into why you think and act the way you do.
- After identifying particular problems or behaviours, you can be taught specific skills and techniques such as mindfulness or CBT to address them. Eclectic therapies help clients identify and replace unhealthy coping strategies with healthier behaviours.
- They do not follow a strict formula or lesson plan like in CBT.

Matching Therapies to Illness

You may have a sense of which of the four approaches is right for you. How do you know what specific therapy to choose? While some therapies are specific to an illness such as trauma, many others, such as CBT, can be applied to a broad range of illnesses. If someone suggests that a certain therapy technique is best for you, how do you know if that's true?

One starting point is asking what therapies are recommended in the *clinical guidelines* for your illness. Clinical guidelines are broad-based consensus documents that gather and evaluate the evidence for various treatments of a particular illness.

As an example, for psychological treatment of acute major depressive disorder, the 2016 CANMAT[1] guidelines recommend the following:

First line (most evidence for effectiveness):

- cognitive behavioural therapy (CBT);
- interpersonal therapy (IPT); and
- behavioural activation (BA).

Second line:

- mindfulness based cognitive therapy (MBCT);
- cognitive-behavioural analysis system of psychotherapy (CBASP);
- problem-solving therapy (PST);
- short-term psychodynamic psychotherapy (STPP);
- telephone-delivered CBT and IPT; and
- internet- and computer-assisted therapy.

Third line:

- long-term psychodynamic psychotherapy (PDT);
- acceptance and commitment therapy (ACT);
- video-conferenced psychotherapy; and
- motivational interviewing (MI).

Most reputable therapists should be able to point you toward relevant clinical guidelines or describe how the treatments they offer fit within those guidelines. It never hurts to ask someone else, such as your family doctor, if the guidelines and the suggested therapy seem legitimate.

You'll find sources to locate guidelines in *Appendix A*, and brief descriptions of many common therapies in *Appendix B*.

Managing Therapy

Talk therapy can be time-consuming and costly. Some people continue in therapy for years on end, with no real improvement. Even if you're working with a skilled therapist, you still want to make sure what you're doing is actually helping.

Managing talk therapy goes back to your living treatment plan. After all, talk therapy is one of several types of interventions to treat your symptoms and accomplish your goals. You may make great progress in therapy. But does it improve your life in the ways that you've identified as important? When deciding to pursue therapy, make sure to answer some key questions:

- What do you hope to achieve from this therapy? What are your goals? How will it improve your current situation? Your ongoing mental health symptoms? How will you know whether it is working?

- What should you expect if you pursue this therapy? What happens during sessions? What about between sessions? How long would it likely take to see changes? How big would any improvement be? Do these fit with your overall treatment goals?

- Can you get the most from this therapy at this point? If learning skills and techniques, are you having concentration problems? If delving into your past, do you have the emotional strength required, or will it just cause you to panic? If not, what else could you do first to prepare?

- Is a good, well-qualified therapist for this type of therapy available? Affordable? A good fit for your particular needs and situation?

- What other treatment options are available to you? Is pursuing this therapy the best option at this time? Can other treatments be pursued at the same time?

Working with a therapist will often span many sessions, over weeks, months, or even years. Identify specific evaluation points. At those times, measure your progress against your goals, expectations, and symptoms. Discuss your progress with your therapist. Don't continue indefinitely with a therapist who no longer meets your needs.

As always, share your treatment plan with your therapist as well as all your other treatment providers. You want everyone to understand your overall goals and how their piece fits into the complete picture.

Summary

- There are hundreds of different types of therapies. They can be delivered individually or in a group, and provided by a range of professionals or none at all.
- We categorize therapies as offering practical advice for current problems, teaching skills or techniques, and depth therapies that explore issues from your past. Most therapists combine these into an eclectic mix to suit their clients.
- Clinical guidelines help identify a set of therapies to consider for a particular illness. Some therapies are more generally applied than others.
- Therapy should be managed in the context of your living treatment plan. What are your goals? How and when will you evaluate your progress?

23

Finding a Therapist

In the previous chapter, you caught a glimpse of the different types of talk therapies available. Not every therapy helps with every problem. Your goal is to find both the therapy and the therapist that will help you. This is not easy. Early in your mental health journey, you may not fully understand or be able to express the problems you're experiencing.

Training, education, and experience can vary widely among therapists. Knowing the basics of mental illness, diagnosis, or any particular therapy is not a given. You hope that if you approach someone who can't help you, they suggest alternatives. That isn't necessarily the case.

This chapter is all about finding a therapist who can help you. They need to understand your situation. You may show up with a diagnosis and clearly identified goals. Or, your therapist may need to help you start from scratch, exploring your symptoms to identify goals.

Having identified the problems, hopefully correctly, they need to confirm the most suitable types of therapy. This may not be straightforward. If a type of therapy is appropriate, hopefully they have the training and experience to provide it. If therapy isn't appropriate or other treatments are better suited, perhaps the therapist can direct you to the right provider.

Types of Therapists

Finding someone to provide talk therapy can be extremely challenging. In most places, anyone can call themselves a counsellor or therapist. Specific qualifications or expertise aren't required. However, most train in disciplines such as psychology or social work. The amount and areas of training can vary. You may be surprised to know that some counsellors, therapists, and psychologists have no training whatsoever in mental illness or knowledge of the DSM, etc. (Thankfully, most do.)

Many people rely on recommendations from others they know and trust. But with the wide variety of people, personalities, problems, and treatments, what works for one person won't necessarily work for you.

If you're looking for a therapist, start with their background and qualifications. We'll discuss three aspects of this: training, the role of regulated professionals, and worldview.

Specific Training

If you're looking for someone to help with diagnosis, look for (or ask them for) evidence that they've received appropriate training. It could have been a major part of a university degree. It could also come from courses or workshops in specific areas. Ask them if they follow the DSM, the role diagnosis would play in your treatment, how they approach therapy, etc.

Similarly, if you're looking to treat a specific problem, ask about their qualifications to treat that problem. Have they received training in relevant therapies? How much training and from where? Ask them why a particular treatment is right for your situation and what the alternatives are. How mainstream is the type of treatment they provide? Can they provide independent, credible evidence that this treatment is appropriate? Run their answers by someone you trust who has some understanding of the area.

Unfortunately, a therapist's degree by itself may not tell you very much. Someone with a BA, MA, or PhD in Psychology may have done most of their coursework in abnormal psychology, i.e., mental illness, which would be helpful. However, instead, they could have trained primarily in experimental psychology, human factors, psychometry, etc. These won't provide enough of the relevant training needed to be a good therapist. The same applies to degrees in social work, education, etc.—all vast areas of study.

Of course, someone with excellent credentials may not be able to help you, while someone with a thinner resume might have the right skills and experience obtained through other means. Personal recommendations and reputation play a big role.

Regulated Professionals

If someone says they are a medical doctor, you can assume they completed standard training and have certain qualifications. Legislation regulates who can call themselves a doctor. Other professional titles may also be regulated in this way. What titles are regulated, and the qualifications needed to use each title, vary widely between jurisdictions.

For example, in Canada, each province has different legislation creating a number of regulated health professions. Each profession creates a regulating body, typically called a *college*, that defines educational requirements, practice standards, and guidelines, as well as disciplinary processes. If someone meets these requirements and agrees to abide by the standards and guidelines (and pays a fee), they can become a member of that specific college. In return, the province provides exclusive use of a professional designation to members of that college.

Legislation only restricts the use of the exact designation. While "Registered Psychologist" may be regulated, if "psychologist" is not, anyone is free to use it. This could be someone who completed a PhD in psychology, someone with an undergrad degree in psychology, or even someone who took one course or read a book on psychology.

A therapist using a regulated professional designation guarantees a level of training. This does not guarantee that they're an appropriate person to help you of course. Other titles or designations, whether backed by a trade organization or made up out of thin air, provide far fewer guarantees.

This doesn't mean that someone without a professional designation can't be very helpful to you. You'll just have to ask more questions to find out. Remember, different jurisdictions have various regulated professional designations, standards, and rules. Do your research.

Worldview

Earlier in the book, we described the biopsychosocial model. Those who subscribe to this model understand mental illness is rooted in a mix of biological, psychological, and social factors. The appropriateness of treatments is determined based on scientific evidence. This model, and the set of perspectives and assumptions behind it, is an example of a *worldview*.

Depending on their background, some people seek out counsellors or therapists whose worldview includes spiritual or religious components. This would include clergy or new age practitioners.

Different worldviews strongly influence the treatments therapists provide and the advice they give. Beware of anyone who doesn't know the limits of what they can provide. They should recommend you see someone else when needed. A responsible priest won't hesitate to direct a suicidal person to their doctor or emergency psychiatric resources rather than performing an exorcism. Psychiatrists and psychologists frequently refer patients to one another, recognizing the limits of what each brings to the table.

Ideally, any provider you see will help you find the right treatment for you, no matter who may deliver it.

Some people who work as counsellors or therapists have a very limited worldview. At the extreme, you'll find people who don't believe that mental illness is real or biologically based, just different ways of seeing the world. We should embrace these differences, not treat them.

Others believe that mental illness is real, but that all cases are due to one cause, e.g., vitamin deficiencies, childhood trauma, sexual abuse, or gender identity. This can go the other way too. Some people feel that medications are always the right choice for mental health issues, never therapy.[1]

Who to Pick

By now, you probably have a few ideas about what you're looking for. Maybe you've read about the regulated professions in your area and narrowed down the type of therapist you'd like to see. You may clearly understand what problem you want addressed or even what type of therapy you're interested in. The more you know about what you need, the easier it will be. Now what? Time to go therapist shopping? Maybe…

Not to put the brakes on rampant consumerism, but you are looking for someone to improve your health. Like any other intervention, make decisions about therapy with your treatment goals, timeframes, and other alternatives top of mind. Consult your living treatment plan, not only when finding a therapist but also periodically to track your progress.

Costs and Other Realities

In an ideal world, you'd be able to see whoever can best meet your needs. But there are practical realities as well. One of the biggest is cost. Some people can afford to pay for therapy out of pocket, but most cannot. Most insurance plans either don't cover therapy or limit the number of sessions they support. Therapy for a substantial problem will generally involve many sessions. With typical rates of $150 per hour and up, it adds up quickly.

The following sections outline resources that may be available to reduce or eliminate the cost. What each offers can vary. Even if you have access to affordable therapy, make sure it suits your needs. Free therapy that doesn't help isn't worth the price.

At the very least, be conscious of the costs when considering your options. There are other practical considerations, such as location and distance. Are there other concerns such as accessibility to worry about? And, of course, is the person you want to see available? Some therapists may have a full practice or have restrictions on who they take as clients.

General Search Tips

If you're working through insurance, an HMO, or your company's EAP, they may have a list of people you can see. Otherwise, where do you begin?

Word of mouth is always a good starting point. Does your doctor or another health professional have anyone they recommend for your situation? Do people in your life who are open about mental health have any recommendations? Always keep in mind their needs may be very different from yours. Even if a friend's fabulous therapist is utterly wrong for you, they may be able to suggest who you should contact.

Most therapists who take private clients also have websites with information about their training, background, types of therapies they use, and problems they see most frequently. If you're interested in seeing someone from one of the regulated health professions in your area, check the website for that professional college. They may have a directory of members or a referral service that helps match your needs with one of their members.

If you've identified a few names, get in touch with them. Many offer a free or low-cost brief consultation, whether via telephone or in person. You can use this conversation to see if they might be a good match. Think about the questions you'd like to ask them ahead of time.

Finally, even if you start working with someone, you're under no obligation to keep working with them. Finding a therapist who can help you involves not only their skills and training but a comfortable personal connection. Don't feel you need to stay with someone if the fit is just not there.

Health Benefits

When it comes to covering the costs of therapy, health insurance plans are one common way to do it. Many people have plans, whether purchased on their own or provided via a government program or their employer.

If you do have health benefits, read your plan brochure carefully. Find out precisely what is and is not covered, as well as any restrictions or constraints. Plans often pay for a fixed number of sessions per year and may cover only part of the rate charged by the therapist. They may place restrictions on who you can see. For example, your plan may only cover $50 per session for up to six therapy sessions a year with a Registered Psychologist.

Employee Assistance Plans

Many companies offer workers therapy through an EAP. Typically, the therapy consists of shorter-term practical advice from counsellors via telephone or face-to-face sessions. You're restricted as to who you see or speak with under this arrangement, though the entire cost is usually covered.

As with psychology coverage in extended health plans, they may limit how many sessions you can use. Unlike extended health plans, there is a bit more flexibility and the possibility of exceptions. After all, companies pay for EAPs to keep their employees at work. If an extra hour or two in therapy will help do that, it's worth it to them.

Remember that EAPs are there to support your continued functioning in the workplace. The type of therapy or support you'll receive is somewhat more limited and practical in nature than if you were paying out of pocket.

Long-Term Disability Insurance

If you are off work for a considerable time, usually 90 days or more, you may be receiving long-term disability (LTD) benefits. If a mental health concern is part of the reason you're unable to work, you may be able to have therapy covered by insurance.

To make this happen, you need to convince your case manager at your LTD provider (insurance company) that therapy would help you return to work sooner. Often, they arrange for you to see a psychologist for a few initial sessions. The psychologist then proposes they cover an extra number of therapy sessions. While the psychologist is often independent, they effectively work for the insurance company. They will report on your progress, identify obstacles preventing you from returning to work, etc.

It may help to ask your family doctor (or psychiatrist, if you have one) to write to the insurance company asking them to fund a psychologist. When you're off work for health reasons, your insurance company is usually in contact with your doctors already. These recommendations can carry some weight with insurance companies, so are worth pursuing.

Sliding Fee Scales

On occasion, the cost of therapy is based on a *sliding scale.* It is adjusted based on your financial situation. Not many therapists are in a position to be able to do this—they need to eat and pay bills, too!

Therapists who charge on a sliding scale may do so within their regular practice. Or, they may volunteer part-time at a clinic where everyone pays either a deeply-discounted or pay-what-you-can rate. If you have trouble locating someone in your area, ask your doctor. They generally know who can provide subsidized counselling or therapy.

Community Clinics

You may have a mental health clinic or other organization in your area that provides some counselling or psychotherapy at no charge. These are generally government funded. Depending on their organizational structure and mandate, they may limit the amount of support they can provide and the types of issues they focus on. You may or may not need a referral from a family doctor to access these clinics.

Doctors?

These days, doctors are generally moving away from small, independent practices. In some areas, family doctors are grouped into team-based practices, either in a single clinic space or linking the services of several clinics in the area. Often with some government funding, they can offer services that are not viable in independent medical practices. Access to mental health workers is one such service. These groups go by different names, such as *primary care networks* or *family health teams.* Ask your family doctor if they have access to any mental health resources connected to their practice.

There are also psychiatrists who do an extensive amount of psychotherapy in their practices. As health insurance plans may cover psychotherapy provided by doctors, this can be very attractive. The downside is that very few psychiatrists provide an extensive amount, and waiting lists are almost always exceptionally long.

Alternatives to Therapists

If you can't afford (or can't find) an individual therapist to provide the type of therapy you need to meet your specific goals, there may be alternatives.

One option is a more affordable therapist in another location. Many offer therapy via Skype or FaceTime. Online brokers are emerging that connect patients with appropriate therapists. Of course, everything we discussed earlier about checking into a therapist's qualifications, background, and type of therapy offered still applies.

If you're looking to learn new skills and techniques (rather than seeking practical advice or a depth therapy), you'll have more options. As we noted, these types of therapies aren't closely tied to your personal situation.

We've already mentioned groups and courses teaching skills such as mindfulness or CBT. You may be able to find no-cost or low-cost options in your area. While not ideal, there are online skills courses, too.

Books can also help you learn skills and techniques. Of particular help are workbooks that provide step-by-step instruction, along with exercises at each step. Many excellent workbooks have been created by leaders in the field who have taught a therapy for many years. You can find some recommendations on our website; see *Appendix A*.

There are also many mental health smartphone apps, though of highly variable quality. Some help teach you a technique and are set up like a book or workbook, though often contain only a small subset of what you'd find elsewhere. Others help you practice a technique once you've learned it. Mood tracker apps allow you to monitor your symptoms and may remind you to practice or guide you through some techniques.

Summary

- Interpreting a therapist's training or credentials is difficult. Some are members of regulated professional colleges.
- Keep in mind constraints such as cost, location, and insurance coverage, but make sure the therapy they offer will meet your needs.
- Group benefits may include employee assistance plans, which can provide some therapy. Extended health benefits may pay for other therapists.
- Some clinics offer fees on a sliding scale based on income. Other more affordable options are therapy groups, courses, workbooks, or apps.

24

The Role of Medications

This chapter introduces psychotropic medications. We'll cover some of the basics, including how they generally work and what they're used for. In the following chapters, we'll look at specific types of medications such as antidepressants in more detail.

There's a large amount of information about medications in this book compared with other types of treatments. This doesn't mean that medications are more important or should be used more often. Rather, medications are some of the most poorly understood, complex, and frequently misused treatments available. At the same time, they are often readily available and can be very effective when used properly.

Let's state the obvious. Recreational use aside, you don't take any medication for the fun of it. You take it because the medical condition it's supposed to treat is harming your health, life, and future. You hope the medication can fix this. Medications have the potential to greatly and quickly improve your mental health. The payoff can be huge, but so are the challenges. Your active involvement, using your living treatment plan, can tilt the odds in your favour and speed up your recovery.

We don't think medications are for everyone, but hope you'll approach these chapters with fresh eyes. We'll do our best to get you up to speed as simply and quickly as possible. Our goal is to deliver a balanced and realistic overview to help you decide if they might have a place in your living treatment plan. Used properly, medications are powerful tools that can help you regain control of your life and improve your functioning. Used improperly, they are, at best, unhelpful, and, at worst, they can lead to many problems.

Medications 101

We'll start with the basics. What are psychotropic medications and how do they work? We'll also discuss why using them correctly is more complicated than using most other medications. People frequently abandon medications that would have improved their health due to some very avoidable mistakes.

Types of Medications

We'll cover five major types of psychotropic medications in the following chapters:

1. *Antidepressants* (e.g., Prozac, Effexor) are what most people think of when psychotropic medications are mentioned. Taken daily, they help with depression of course, but also anxiety and other conditions.
2. *Sedatives and hypnotics* (e.g., Valium, Ativan) help to quickly calm people down during stressful events. Some treat insomnia or are used until an antidepressant starts working.
3. *Mood stabilizers* (e.g., lithium, Epival) are most often used to smooth out the highs (mania) and lows experienced by people with bipolar disorders, but they can help people diagnosed with depression, too.
4. *Antipsychotics* (e.g., Seroquel, Risperdal) are used to treat psychosis in people with schizophrenia or in a manic episode. At lower doses, they complement other treatments for many mental illnesses.
5. *Stimulants* (e.g., Ritalin, Adderall) help people with Attention-Deficit Hyperactivity Disorder, treat fatigue, and improve concentration.

How They Work

As we describe different medications, we'll give you a basic overview of not only what they are used for, but also the neuroscience explaining how each medication works. It won't surprise you that most medications affect the transmission of neurotransmitters (serotonin, norepinephrine, dopamine, GABA, glutamate, and others to lesser degrees).

Medication Selection

There are dozens of different psychotropic medications. Predicting which one will work best with reasonable certainty is currently impossible. With many physical illnesses, after a quick exam or lab test, a doctor can prescribe a medication they know will probably help, such as an antibiotic for an infection. Unfortunately, mental health medications are more unpredictable. The science isn't there yet.

You may have to try several medications to find one that works. If the first one didn't work (or caused side effects), don't conclude that psychotropic medications aren't right for you. Similarly, because a medication was amazingly helpful for someone you know, don't be disappointed if it doesn't help you. If you're going to try psychotropic medications, expect some trial and error.

Is picking the right medication simply guessing at random? Not at all. Doctors take into account many factors when selecting a medication for you to try. Your symptoms will guide them to a class of medications based on which neurotransmitters need to be targeted. Other symptoms tell them to stay away from medications targeting other neurotransmitters. How you've tolerated and responded to other medications also influences the decision. Genetics play a significant role, so if a close relative responded well to a medication there's a greater chance you will too. Chronic health conditions raise the risk of some medications or make them less effective. Interactions with other medications or supplements can be a concern. Then there are issues such as cost, how and when the medication needs to be taken, how long it lasts, and more. Your doctor tries to keep up with all the new medications and lessons about existing ones, but it's not easy.

Psychotropic medications operate on molecules, which then change how billions of electrical signals are transmitted. Depending on the pattern of signals, a change in mood occurs. The complexity makes it difficult to predict what medications will work. While genetic testing and advanced imaging can help somewhat, these tests are expensive and not in wide use. Researchers are busy working on other tools to make better predictions.

Expectations

Most people don't know what to expect when first prescribed a psychotropic medication. These medications often behave differently than other medications. For example, most antidepressants take weeks before you experience any effect. Many psychotropics are started below the effective dose so you can physically get used to them. If you aren't told these things, it is normal to feel frustrated when you are not cured in a few days or weeks. Even medication side effects can be different because neurotransmitters are found in both your brain and other areas of your body. If nobody tells you what to expect, what to be concerned about, and what will likely disappear over time, you're more likely to stop taking a medication long before it's had a chance to work.

In this and the following chapters, you'll learn what to expect from different types of medications. You'll also learn the questions you need to ask and some ways you can find answers to your questions.

How Can Medications Help?

What problems can medications help with? Certainly not everything. They won't help with relationship problems, unhealthy coping, or physical illness causing mental health symptoms. Even then, they can manage some symptoms, but you'll need something else to fix the underlying problem.

Severe Illness

Most people with severe mental illness, e.g., schizophrenia, need medications for daily functioning. Without them, they lose touch with reality, hearing or seeing things that aren't there. They may believe they have superpowers or that the CIA has infiltrated their home. People suffering from severe depression need medication to decrease long-term suicidal thoughts. All of these have dangerous consequences.

Medications provide the stability needed for good self-care, to go to work or school, and maintain relationships. Other tools, such as psychotherapy, may help a bit, but, without medication, are not sufficient. While people with severe mental illness also have serious difficulties accessing effective care, their experiences, needs, and struggles are often very different than those of the people we expect to read this book.

Improve Short-Term Functioning

Medications are often used to help get you back on your feet again. When you are depressed or anxious, they decrease your anxiety each morning, help you get out of bed, and prevent a panic attack. Medications help you regain your independence, so you rely less on friends and family. They improve your concentration and performance at work.

You may be faced with new stressors or have skeletons in your closet. You may have experienced some form of abuse, a chaotic family environment, a recent loss, or something that you know has deeply affected you. But, now is not the right time to deal with those problems. You know that medication can't fix them, but it can shut off the worry so you can function well and meet your commitments.

People often seek treatment for mental health problems when they're in the middle of a crisis. They have severe problems that are affecting them right now. Medication can be an effective tool to help end the crisis.

Emotional Resilience

Like most people, you probably have had difficult experiences involving your relationships, your jobs, or in your childhood. Do you have enough emotional muscle to deal with them?

Counselling and psychotherapy can help you recognize problematic patterns of behaviour. You can then learn techniques or find new ways to deal with stressful situations. This takes a lot of hard work, learning new things, and practicing. You're essentially rewiring your brain, replacing unhelpful behaviours and habits with healthier ones.

If you're in crisis, you probably don't have the emotional resilience needed to benefit from psychotherapy. You won't grasp the techniques or retain what you've learned. You may be too scared or not have the energy to practice the skills. If you have a panic attack every time your therapist mentions an event from your past, you're not going to get far.

In these situations, medications can help. They calm you down and increase your motivation and concentration. They build up your emotional armour so that you can handle the stresses that therapy brings. Sure, it's a band-aid, but you may need to stop the bleeding before you can get to fixing the underlying problem.

After you've learned new habits, behaviours, and coping strategies, you may find that you don't need the medications anymore. You can then be weaned off them if you and your treatment providers feel it makes sense. It's important to follow your doctor's instructions when stopping psychotropic medications. This is discussed in the following chapters.

It's common for people to see multiple mental health providers. A psychiatrist might prescribe medications for you and a psychologist might provide psychotherapy. Each plays a different but necessary role in your treatment. It's the combination that helps you reach wellness.

Long-Term Symptom Management

Medications can also be used long term. They aren't only used when you are in crisis or when you need more resilience for psychotherapy. For many people, medications are a sensible approach to treatment over the long term. It seems almost ludicrous having to say that. Most people don't feel a need to justify taking insulin if they have diabetes, taking anticonvulsants if they have epilepsy, or taking blood pressure medications for hypertension, even if it's for the rest of their life.

Often, several different treatment approaches would be sensible. It then becomes a matter of weighing the costs and benefits of each. Some people find that medication is the most practical way to manage their symptoms. If taking a pill each day keeps you well, that's pretty convenient.

Why Medications Are Used

We know what psychotropic medications are and what kind of mental health problems they are ideally suited for. We now want to turn to a slightly different question: why are they used?

In other words, if you've got several different tools to pick from that might reasonably address your symptoms, e.g., medication and counselling, why might you choose medication? It's not always because medication is the best tool for the job.

Effectiveness

Medications are used to treat mental health problems because they work. That is, when an appropriate medication is used to help with an appropriate problem, it has been shown to be very effective. Compared with many medical treatments, that means if your doctor starts you on a psychotropic medication, there's a very good chance (albeit with a bit of trial and error) that medication will help.

How effective are psychotropics compared to other medications? One way to compare is by asking how many people you'd need to give the medication to before you saw a positive result. That would be "10" if on average one out of ten people saw a result, and "1" if everyone saw a result.[1]

To prevent one heart attack with low-dose aspirin: *1,500-2,000*

To prevent one heart attack with statins: *40-100*

To prevent a second seizure with anti-epileptic medications: *10*

To recover from depression with antidepressants: *4*

Yes, *four!* This shows antidepressants are incredibly effective. Studies for various types of psychotropics and appropriate illnesses frequently show numbers in the single digits.

Yet, some people who have tried one or more medications haven't found them helpful. Sometimes this is a result of an incorrect diagnosis, missing other problems, or completely inappropriate medication choices. More often, this happens when medication trials aren't run well. We'll talk more about this later.

Accessibility and Affordability

Limited access to alternatives is one reason that medication may be used more than other treatments. At times, they are used for problems they really aren't intended to solve.

Accessibility comes down to the issue of providers' availability, time, and resources. If you go to your family doctor for help with mental health, you're more likely to leave with a prescription. Consider the alternatives. They don't have the time to provide you with extensive psychotherapy. Trying to connect you with the right therapist is difficult and time-consuming, particularly if you're on a tight budget. Helping with complex issues is impractical during a short doctor's appointment.

Being able to afford treatment plays a huge role in being able to access it. In places such as Canada, everyone can visit a family doctor at no cost. In contrast, professionals such as psychologists aren't generally covered by basic health insurance. Unless you're lucky enough to have a publicly funded clinic available with the services you need, you may not be able to pay for treatment.

Coverage for the cost of medications varies, too. For example, Canada has universal healthcare but not universal pharmacare. Paying for medications often costs less than paying for therapy. Depending on the medication, a month's worth of medication could cost the equivalent of ten minutes of therapy.

Without the cash to pay for medication, there are usually a few options:

- Employer or other group benefits programs often have medication coverage.
- Some provincial or state governments offer for-fee group benefit plans open to anyone in that province.
- For those with somewhat lower income, some governments have programs that cap the amount you have to pay for medication.
- For those who are very low income, social assistance programs may provide some form of medication coverage.
- Many pharmaceutical companies offer compassionate programs and can provide their specific medication to people who need it, but who can't afford it and can't access other programs.

> - Pharmaceutical sales reps often give samples to doctors to make it easier to try people on their medication. Sometimes they can provide enough samples to "float" one or more patients long term.
>
> If you're having trouble paying for medication, talk to your doctor about it. They may not know the price of the medication they are prescribing. They may be able to prescribe similar alternatives that are more affordable. Your pharmacist will be able to tell you what different medications cost. They may know of programs that you are eligible for that could reduce the cost.

Your Time and Effort

We started this chapter by saying that nobody takes medication for fun. Taking medication is a better option than doing nothing to improve your health. There are things that many people like even less than taking a medication. Depending on the person, these might include

- spending hours in therapy confronting uncomfortable thoughts and feelings;
- engaging in increasingly scary activities to overcome a fear or phobia;
- reading and practicing techniques from a workbook; and
- exercising, eating healthier, or cutting back on caffeine or alcohol.

Let's face it: a lot of people either don't have the time or would rather do other things with their time. They would rather take a pill each day.

Controversies, Conspiracies, and Concerns

If you haven't already, you'll likely encounter a few people with strong negative feelings about psychotropic medications and, often, psychiatry as a whole.

Some people may tell you all mental health problems are overreactions. They do not represent illness. Or, they may say that people who rely on medication are too lazy to eat well and exercise. They're just not trying hard enough. That's nonsense!

Many of these people have had bad personal experiences. Some may have even been given potent medications against their will while involuntarily committed to a hospital. You'll find these individuals gathered in psychiatric survivor groups. Some identify as anti-psychiatry and hold the extreme view that the field of psychiatry should be abolished. The internet has given these people a louder voice.

There are legitimate concerns associated with taking any medication. But when people start telling you that "mental illness isn't real," medications are a means of "state control," and that it's all a profit-driven scheme by "Big Pharma" to get you addicted, they're crossing the line between legitimate concern and paranoid conspiracy.

Yes, pharmaceutical companies have more influence than they probably should. Understanding of some of the underlying neurobiological mechanisms is still advancing. And, involuntary psychiatric treatment for extreme circumstances is never ideal. We're not discounting skepticism, but it has to have some basis in a broad-based reality.

We want to caution you that when people share their experiences, remember that their circumstances are not necessarily yours. Everyone is different, especially when it comes to mental health. Be wary of all-or-nothing views, regardless of the source. If you have concerns, speak with your doctor or other mental health professionals.

Should You Consider Medications?

As with any health issue, learn as much as you can in order to help improve your mental health. Consider any credible, evidence-based treatment that is appropriate for your circumstances. Choose the ones that best meet your own unique needs. Any treatment decisions will involve trade offs, costs, and benefits. Remember that neglecting your symptoms has costs, too.

We've already stated that medications may help with certain problems but not others. They may assist you in getting the most out of other treatments such as psychotherapy. But before looking at any lengthy treatment, ruling out other physical causes of your symptoms (as we discussed in the *Physical Illness* chapter) is a must.

For many with mild to moderate anxiety or depression, lifestyle choices can have a similar impact to an antidepressant. And there are countless other benefits of regular exercise, improving your diet, getting proper sleep, and cutting back on alcohol and caffeine that we've talked about previously.

It's not unusual to try improving lifestyle choices to see if your symptoms improve. You can then decide whether adding medication makes sense. Some people choose to forego alternatives if they are available and prefer to take medication. Your illness, goals, and timeframes may influence your choices. There's no right or wrong answer.

Medications, used well, can be a useful part of your overall treatment. We hope this and the following chapters help you make an informed choice.

> ### Summary
>
> - Psychotropic medications include antidepressants, sedatives and hypnotics, mood stabilizers, antipsychotics, and stimulants.
>
> - Psychotropics work on neurotransmitters and can take time before they start working. Side effects when starting are common. Finding the right medication often involves some trial and error, but a good trial takes time.
>
> - Medications can help with severe mental illness, improve short-term functioning, build emotional resilience to help with psychotherapy, or provide long-term symptom management.
>
> - Despite conspiracy theories to the contrary, psychotropics can be effective and affordable options. They may be the only effective option for some situations or one of several treatment options, each with benefits and risks.

25

Antidepressants

Now that we've talked about psychotropic medications in general, let's get a bit more specific. This chapter covers antidepressants, which constitutes a broad and varied category of medications.

Antidepressants are far more complicated to take than medications you may be familiar with. How do they work? What do they help with? What should you expect? How long do you take them for? The answers are not always straightforward, leaving many people mystified. Suboptimal use is widespread.

Broadly speaking, the many antidepressants are more similar than different. Understanding what they have in common is 90% of the battle. You'll learn all about that here. For the last 10%, *Appendix C* briefly describes individual antidepressants, pointing out what makes each one unique.

By the end of this chapter, you'll better understand when antidepressants are used, when they shouldn't be used, and how they work. You'll also learn how you and your doctor can select specific antidepressants for your particular situation. Most importantly, if you do try an antidepressant, you'll make smart decisions and have a realistic idea of what to expect.

Uses

Despite the name, antidepressants are not only used for depression. They treat many mental health disorders. They are the preferred medications for most forms of anxiety, obsessive-compulsive disorders, trauma, impulsivity, and some eating disorders, to name a few. They are used for several non-mental health issues, including pain management and even irritable bowel syndrome.

Bipolar Disorder

If you're considering taking an antidepressant, read this carefully. Antidepressants are used only with extreme caution if you are prone to episodes of hypomania or mania, which are hallmarks of bipolar disorders. If depressive episodes are periods of very low mood, hypomania and mania are periods of very high mood and energy. According to the DSM-5, these episodes include at least three of the following symptoms:

1. Inflated self-esteem or grandiosity.
2. Decreased need for sleep (e.g., rested after 3 hours of sleep).
3. More talkative than usual or pressure to keep talking.
4. Racing thoughts or rapidly shifting between ideas (e.g., rambling).
5. Easily distracted by unimportant or irrelevant things.
6. Increase in school/work/social activities, or purposeless physical movements driven by mental agitation (e.g., pacing, wringing hands).
7. Engaging in uncharacteristically high-risk activities (e.g., excessive shopping sprees, sexual practices or relationships).

Full-blown mania will disrupt your life and you may need hospitalization. Hypomania isn't as severe but still a substantial change from normal. It's not just a good day. Have you ever had an episode that sounds like this? Did it last most of the day for at least a few days? Tell your doctor, even if it was triggered by medications or illicit drugs. You may have a bipolar disorder or be more prone to hypomania or mania than most people.

Doctors prescribing antidepressants should ask about hypomania or mania, though sometimes this is little more than, "Have you ever spent too much money?" If you suspect past hypomania or mania, speak up, even if you're not asked. If you are prone to such episodes, an antidepressant increases the risk of another episode. This can happen even if you only had one hypomanic episode twenty years ago. Even if you're now struggling purely with depression, an antidepressant may not be the right choice. Other medications such as mood stabilizers may be more appropriate.

People who have had hypomania or mania can take antidepressants. It is almost always in combination with a mood stabilizer or other medication. Such a regime is also usually started only under the close supervision of a psychiatrist.

> Everyone with a bipolar disorder is different. Some people are primarily depressed and had a single hypomanic episode years ago. Others develop hypomania or mania much more frequently. Using an antidepressant is riskier in the second group than the first, though both groups are at far greater risk than people who have never had such an episode.
>
> The fear of using antidepressants in anyone with a history of bipolar disorders can go to an extreme. We've seen several people who carried a diagnosis of a bipolar disorder for decades. Unfortunately, they only had one episode, which didn't actually meet the criteria for hypomania or mania. The episode wasn't as severe as once thought, didn't last more than a short time, or illicit substances were involved (even if they didn't admit it at the time).
>
> We've also seen people labelled bipolar for dozens of years who had seen several psychiatrists. Skeptical, we obtained and carefully reviewed their previous medical records. The first psychiatrist they saw noted "rule out possible bipolar" in their report. That is doctor-speak meaning they didn't have time to confirm or exclude it. The second read the first note and, based solely on that, diagnosed "possible bipolar." The third read the second note and diagnosed "bipolar by history." The fourth read the third note and diagnosed the definitive sounding "bipolar." This diagnosis was then carried forward indefinitely. This all happened without further discussion or investigation of any past episodes.
>
> Carrying around such a false bipolar diagnosis can affect your current treatment. Avoiding antidepressants may be a tremendous missed opportunity. If something about a longstanding diagnosis doesn't ring true, try to get a hold of your previous records. You never know what they might reveal.

How They Work

Like most psychotropic medications, antidepressants affect neurotransmitters. Most often they affect one or more ways of transmitting serotonin (5-HT), norepinephrine (NE), and dopamine (DA).

They use a variety of different mechanisms to influence this transmission. For example, the most common class of medications today are Selective Serotonin Reuptake Inhibitors (SSRIs). As the name suggests, they inhibit (reduce) reuptake of serotonin from the synapse into the nerve's axon. This increases the chance of binding to serotonin receptors and thus improves signal transmission. Many antidepressants use more than one mechanism and affect more than one neurotransmitter.

Medications within the same class may have similarities but are not interchangeable. And, of course, there are many classes of antidepressants.

What to Expect

For most people, an antidepressant can be one of the most confusing medications they've ever taken. Let's discuss step by step what you need to know.

Start-Up and Dosing

Antidepressants need to be started at a low dose and slowly increased. This gives your body time to adjust and minimizes side effects. The starting dose and increment vary between medications, but increases are typically at least a week apart. Otherwise, side effects can be more severe and distressing. Starting at too high a dose or increasing too rapidly are major reasons why antidepressants are stopped prematurely. Like many people, you may have decided that you can't tolerate a medication after a day or two. This may not have happened if you started lower and slower. Unless told otherwise, you assumed the side effects you first experienced would continue as long as you took the medication. However, this is rarely the case, as we'll discuss shortly.

Some antidepressants won't have any effect on your symptoms until they reach at least their target dose. The target dose is usually a range, e.g., 20–50 mg. This means that most people who have their symptoms fully relieved by the medication need a dose within that range. This dose varies greatly between medications, so comparing doses of different antidepressants is like comparing apples and oranges. Finding the right dose can be tricky. Too low and the antidepressant only partially helps. Too high and you may have more side effects than you need to experience. It also takes time. Increasing a week at a time may be enough to minimize side effects. It takes longer, typically four to six weeks at a given dose, to feel the full effect. Too many people give up on medications long before they've had a chance to work.

Most antidepressants have a recommended dosing schedule, specified in the product monograph (the prescribing information given to doctors). Actual practice often differs. And some individuals are more sensitive to medications. They may need an even lower starting dose, and smaller and slower increments. Most antidepressants have a preferred, once-daily extended-release version. Sedating antidepressants are usually taken at night, and more stimulating ones in the morning. If you find a normally sedating one is stimulating, adjust the time accordingly. You may find that instead of one large dose a day, you have fewer side effects if you split your total dose into two small doses taken at different times.

Too many doctors are unable (or unwilling) to spend the time needed to explain all this when they first prescribe you an antidepressant. If you don't know what to expect, you're far more likely to suffer as a result.

> What does starting an antidepressant look like in practice? Consider the typical dosing regime for the antidepressant sertraline (Zoloft). It has a target dose of 50–200 mg for depression.
>
> 1. Your doctor starts you at 25 mg (below the target dose).
> 2. After one week they increase your dose to 50 mg.
> 3. They want to see how you'd do at the low end of the dose range, so they keep you on the 50 mg for four weeks.
> 4. After four weeks at 50 mg, how much did your symptoms improve?
>
> - Worse? It's not likely this will be a good medication for you. They'll drop your dose to 25 mg for a week and then have you stop it and try something else.
> - Close to 100% improvement? That's the dose for you, so no need for further increases.
> - Mostly improved? You're probably close to the right dose. They'll increase to 75 mg, wait another four weeks, and evaluate again.
> - Somewhat improved (i.e., at least 30%)? Odds are the medication will likely help, but you're not close to the right dose yet. They'll increase to 75 mg for one week, and then 100 mg. After four weeks at 100 mg, evaluate again.
> - If 100 mg is very close, they'll bump it up to 125 mg, wait four weeks, and evaluate that.
> - Or, if 100 mg is better but still well below 100%, they'll increase it to 125 mg for one week, then 150 mg, wait four weeks, and evaluate that. They'll repeat if needed until you reach the maximum 200 mg.
>
> This can vary. For example, say your symptoms are more severe, or you've needed doses at the high end of the target range with other antidepressants. Your doctor may increase it weekly by 25 mg until you hit 100 mg or even 150 mg before pausing for several weeks and evaluating. It's a trade-off. On the one hand, you may feel better more quickly. On the other hand, you may overshoot the correct dose. You may have too many side effects and need to backtrack.

Effectiveness

Knowing whether an antidepressant is helping is trickier than most people think. First, the effect builds up slowly, usually over several weeks at a given dose. Second, it may be difficult to notice your improvement or to quantify the gains you've made. Gradual changes are harder to describe than sudden ones. On top of all that, you may have difficulty recalling how you used to feel. This can be caused by your illness itself.

Periodically repeating self-report scales (or using mood tracking apps) may help. They allow you to rate your symptoms over the last week and then compare with previous times you used the scale. Keeping your eye on two or three symptoms that you find particularly bothersome is a more personalized variation. Journalling your symptoms is another approach. Asking family members or others who have spent ample time with you is particularly useful. They usually see changes before you do and can better describe the before and after differences.

Finally, some symptoms tend to improve before others. Problems with fatigue, sleep, and appetite usually improve first. A change in your mood follows. Cognitive and memory deficits can take two or three times as long.

If you're taking an antidepressant to help with anxiety, you may need a higher dose of medication than used to treat depression. It may also take considerably longer before you notice an improvement in your symptoms.

The usual goal of treatment is to remove all symptoms, whether by medication alone or a combination of interventions. This lets you heal and increases your resilience. If symptoms are only partially treated, you'll still be constantly fighting your illness. That makes it more likely you'll experience a recurrence of all your symptoms if you try to stop your treatment. That, in turn, can result in your illness returning full force, and you, ultimately, experiencing another episode with a decline in function and well-being.

One fear that many people have is that antidepressants fundamentally change who they are as a person. Rest assured, this does not happen.

You may find yourself less prone to dark thoughts, or, when they occur, find it easier to get your mind off them. You may no longer have a panic attack when entering a crowded room. You may still be anxious, but not so anxious that you're overwhelmed and can't think. Medications can help take the edge off or make it easier for you to break free from an emotional spiral. They do not change your beliefs, your values, your personality, or anything else that makes you *you*.

While on some medications, you might find that you don't feel as sad, happy, or excited as you were before you were sick. This is known as *emotional numbing*. You may find it harder to think through certain problems than in the past, i.e., brain fog. These are side effects and should be identified and managed working with your doctor.

Side Effects

As with all medications, you may experience side effects when taking an antidepressant. The neurotransmitters that regulate your mood control many other systems throughout your body. Side effects are caused by antidepressants affecting neurotransmitters and receptors in all those areas. Some people have no side effects, some have one or two mild effects for a couple of days, and others have severe side effects that don't go away. Some side effects worsen with higher medication doses. The chance that you will experience a specific side effect differs with each antidepressant. As well, the side effects you experience may be very different than those experienced by a friend on the same medication. It's not easy to predict.

Side effects can include headache, nausea, dizziness, sweating, itching, tremors, brain fog, poor memory, word-finding difficulties, change in sleep patterns, agitation, constipation, diarrhea, decreased libido, or sexual dysfunction. There are others as well. But, just because a medication may cause a side effect doesn't mean that you will experience it.

Timing is very important. Side effects primarily occur when first starting a medication and in the few days after the dose increases. Most ease up and disappear after a few days, occasionally lasting up to a few weeks. If they last any longer than that, they're more likely to persist as long as you're taking that medication.

Stopping an antidepressant when first experiencing a troublesome side effect is one of the most frequent missteps people make. If you are anxious about taking medication, you may focus on a mild side effect that you otherwise could easily tolerate. Be prepared. Try to start your medication when you don't need to be at your best for a few days. Don't overreact. Learn which side effects need to be acted on quickly. For others, try to stick it out a bit. Most of the time, waiting is the answer.

We'll discuss how to deal with many specific side effects in a later chapter. There will also be information about identifying which side effects need urgent attention and which are annoying but harmless.

Stopping

Unless you're on a tiny dose, don't stop antidepressants cold turkey. Just like starting them, decreasing or stopping needs to be done slowly and in small steps. Otherwise, you're very likely to experience withdrawal symptoms, not unlike the side effects we described previously.

Some antidepressants have worse withdrawal symptoms than others. A few, such as venlafaxine (Effexor) and paroxetine (Paxil), leave your system quickly when stopped. Many people experience severe withdrawal with them and even notice if they're a few hours late taking a pill. Others, such as fluoxetine (Prozac), leave your system gradually, minimizing withdrawal. In fact, fluoxetine is often added to smooth out the withdrawal symptoms when stopping other antidepressants. A medication's half-life is a measure of how quickly it leaves your system. Most antidepressants stay in your system for around two weeks, though fluoxetine stays for around seven weeks.

We said the goal of antidepressant treatment is to resolve all symptoms. Then what? If you're taking it for depression, current guidelines[1] suggest after a first episode you should remain on the medication, at the dose leading to wellness, for at least six to nine months after symptoms have fully resolved. For those with more risk factors, such as having had more than one depressive episode or having a chronic physical illness, at least two years is recommended. For those at high risk, having had multiple, severe episodes, an even greater period is probably wise. Discuss when to stop your medication with your doctor. We recommend it be done at an optimal time of year (many people find their mood is best in summer) and during a period of minimal personal stress (no significant life changes about to occur). Some people remain on medication long term. Discuss the benefits and risks of this with your doctor.

Selecting a Medication

If you've glanced at the list of individual antidepressants in *Appendix C*, you know there are many to choose from. That list covers only the most common ones. Around one third of patients find success on the first one they try. We've already said that finding the right one will involve some aspect of trial and error. But this is far from a random process. Many factors can help select the medications most likely to work.

Personal and Family Successes

The first thing to consider is: have you taken an antidepressant before, especially in a similar situation, and found it helpful? Trying that same medication or a very similar one would be a good bet. Similar medications may work on the same neurotransmitters and receptors. They can even be *patent extenders*. These are slightly tweaked versions of a medication released as a new product. They often come with improved side effect profiles.

Mental illness has a strong genetic component to it. If you've had close biological family members who've taken medications, try to find out which ones. Other things being equal, if a family member had success with a medication, you're also likely to.

Symptom Mapping

Next, consider your specific symptoms. Different symptoms are correlated with specific neurotransmitters (5-HT, NE, DA). See Table 25.1.

Table 25.1: Neurotransmitters and symptoms of depression.

Symptom	5-HT	NE	DA
Depressed mood	X	X	X
Psychomotor agitation or retardation	X	X	X
Sleep disturbances	X	X	X
Cognitive problems		X	X
Apathy/loss of interest		X	X
Fatigue		X	X
Guilt/worthlessness	X		
Suicidal ideation	X		
Weight/appetite changes	X		

Let's see how you or your doctor might use this information:

- Your main symptom is a depressed mood. Looking at the table, that can be affected by any of 5-HT, NE, DA, or a combination. That doesn't give you much information about what antidepressant to try.
- If your main symptoms are low motivation and fatigue, a purely serotonergic antidepressant would not be an ideal first choice.
- If you suffer from apathy, poor memory, and weight changes, you'll likely need an antidepressant that targets all three neurotransmitters.

In practice, it's a lot more complicated. There are many more symptoms, such as anxiety and pain, that are affected by these same neurotransmitters. Let's add anxiety and ADHD-like symptoms into the mix, as in Table 25.2.

Table 25.2: Changing neurotransmitters affects other symptoms.

Symptom	↑5-HT	↓5-HT	↑NE	↓NE	↑DA	↓DA
Anxiety	better	worse	worse	better	worse	better
Concentration	–	–	better	worse	better	worse
Attention	–	–	better	worse	–	–

This tells us a few things:

- Antidepressants that increase 5-HT activity improve anxiety. They should be the first choice if your primary symptom is anxiety.
- Increased NE activity helps with some depressive symptoms. It can also make anxiety *worse* but help attention and concentration. With help from your doctor, you may find the right dose of an antidepressant that gives you the best balance between 5-HT and NE.
- More DA activity also worsens anxiety. Unfortunately, stimulants used for ADHD primarily increase DA. Those with anxiety and ADHD need to balance medications to manage all their symptoms.
- Antidepressants that work on NE and DA (e.g., bupropion) can increase anxiety. If you're already anxious, they're more likely to make this worse, not better.

Family doctors who use few antidepressants, and do so less frequently, often don't thoroughly consider symptom mapping. Psychiatrists may do symptom mapping intuitively. Going through the exercise of explicitly identifying which neurotransmitters your symptoms are affected by may serve as an extra check on medication choice. If you find discrepancies, don't jump to conclusions about your medication, but discuss them with your doctor.

Secondary Actions

An antidepressant's main job is to work on depression or anxiety, and each one uses different neurotransmitters and receptors to do that. Because those are found throughout the body, each antidepressant also affects other systems. When those effects are troublesome, you call them side effects. But sometimes these secondary actions can be put to good use.

You can take advantage of secondary actions to help with not only your mood but also another physical problem. For example, some antidepressants (e.g., nortriptyline, duloxetine) are effective at treating some nerve pain. The antidepressant bupropion is effective at smoking cessation (the company that makes the brand-name version, Wellbutrin, also markets the same medication as Zyban for quitting smoking). Some antidepressants, e.g., trazodone, are very sedating, so can be effective in treating insomnia. Others, e.g., mirtazapine, can lead to increased appetite and weight gain and decreased nausea. That is not usually a good thing, but excellent if depression or another illness has resulted in low appetite, nausea, and weight loss.

Metabolism and Interactions

Another factor to consider is how your body absorbs medications. Most are first broken down into small pieces in the gastrointestinal system. The liver then metabolizes them into the form the nervous system needs. It does so using a related set of enzymes, which assist with chemical reactions. There are a dozen different enzymes commonly involved, and most antidepressants use one or more. If an enzyme needed by a medication isn't working well, less will be absorbed by your system, and it will be less effective. These enzymes also transform medications into waste products so they can be removed from the body. Problems can lead to a buildup of medication in your system or a too rapid removal, so it doesn't have time to work.

These enzymes are a common source of medication interactions. If two medications use the same enzyme, an increase or decrease in the amount of either medication in your system can result. This can be dangerous. The same enzymes are affected by many illicit drugs, herbal supplements, and even some foods, such as grapefruit juice.

There are many other reasons medications shouldn't be used together or shouldn't be used if you have some medical conditions. Even future medical issues may need to be taken into account. Thinking of getting pregnant? Some antidepressants are associated with birth defects, while others have been studied extensively and found to be very safe in pregnancy.

> Both your doctor and your pharmacist should keep an eye out for dangerous medication interactions. It's vital that they know everything you're taking, both prescription medications and herbal supplements.
>
> There are interaction checkers on consumer-oriented websites such as rxlist.com and drugs.com. You type in a list of medications, and the site provides a list of possible interactions. These need to be interpreted by your doctor, who would consider your specific health situation, doses of each medication, and more. A particular interaction may or may not apply to you.
>
> Considering interactions doesn't stop once you've chosen an antidepressant. They may be a factor with any medications you add in future.
>
> The liver enzymes described above are part of a class known as *cytochrome P450,* and the reactions they assist are called cytochrome P450 *pathways.* To find out which metabolize a medication or supplement, do an internet search for "CYP450" plus the name of the product.
>
> Interestingly, scientists have found several gene mutations that reduce how well particular pathways work. Ethnic background also affects cytochrome metabolism. Some people already use data from consumer

> genetics testing, e.g., 23andMe, as a factor in medication selection. For example, they avoid medications absorbed by a pathway if they have the relevant mutations. Expect to see more of this in future.

Other Considerations

This section touches on a few more things to be aware of when taking antidepressants. Many are important or serious but will affect very few people.

Suicide Risk

All antidepressants carry a warning that they may increase the risk of suicidal thinking, feeling, or behaviour in children, adolescents, and, to a lesser degree, adults 18–24, in the initial months of treatment. While the risk is very small, the warning is there due to the severity of the consequences.

Depression itself carries a (much higher) risk of suicidal thoughts and actions. So, what's going on here? Several factors may be at work. Antidepressants take weeks to work, and symptoms improve at different rates. If you're depressed and suicidal, you may not have the energy or motivation to act on your thoughts. An antidepressant may boost your energy and motivation long before addressing your thoughts, enabling you to carry out your suicide plan. Second, side effects such as agitation, insomnia, or restlessness can worsen an existing situation. Side effects occur long before the medication has any positive impact. Finally, antidepressants can push people prone to bipolar into a manic state, which carries a higher risk of suicide.

These very small risks can be decreased by thorough history taking and smart prescribing practices. Close monitoring (by you, your doctor, and friend or family supports) is advised when starting any new medication.

Thoughts of suicide are a common symptom of many mental illnesses. They may come and go, and their intensity may vary. Just like other symptoms, don't hesitate to talk with your care providers about these thoughts. Don't be afraid that you'll be locked up just for mentioning it.

Poop-Out Effect

It's common to need small dose adjustments of an antidepressant over time. They could come from more or less stress in your life, or changes in physical health, diet, exercise, or other medications. Sometimes though, you might be on a medication for a few years. With no other changes that you're aware of, the effectiveness of the antidepressant may decrease.

You might question why your mood has changed so drastically when nothing else has. Often, you and your doctor can find something that's changed, e.g., via blood work. If not, it may be that your medication has stopped working for you. You may need to increase your dose, or less commonly, start a different antidepressant to replace it.

Stopping and Restarting

Most people don't want to stay on a medication any longer than they need to. Sometimes people stop to see how they feel without it, taking a so-called *medication holiday*. There is a small chance that if you stop an antidepressant and then later start again, it won't work as well as it did previously.

Serotonin Syndrome

Most antidepressants boost serotonin transmission. Too much of a boost can lead to a potentially dangerous condition called *serotonin syndrome*.[2] It very rarely results from taking two or more serotonergic medications (or much higher than the maximum dose of one). If you are taking a serotonergic antidepressant, be aware that many medications, over-the-counter and natural supplements, and illicit drugs also boost serotonin (see Table 25.3).

Table 25.3: Partial list of substances that boost serotonin levels.

Most antidepressants (all classes)	Opioids (e.g., codeine)
Some mood stabilizers (e.g., lithium)	Stimulants (e.g., Ritalin)
Triptans (used for migraine)	Some muscle relaxants
Some nausea meds (e.g., ondansetron)	Tryptophan, 5-HTP
LSD, Ecstasy, cocaine, methamphetamine	St. John's Wort
Dextromethorphan (in cough syrup)	Panax ginseng
Some antibiotics (e.g., linezolid)	SAMe
Some antipsychotics (e.g., risperidone)	Nutmeg

Symptoms commonly occur within 24 hours of starting a new serotonergic medication or increasing the dose of one you're taking. They can include confusion, agitation, sweating, pupil dilation, headache, involuntary twitching, tremor, palpitations, fever, nausea or vomiting, bruising, hypervigilance, pressured speech, and muscle rigidity. While some of these overlap the side effects that can occur when starting or changing doses of some medications, if you experience several of them (all starting within 24 hours of a new medication or dose increase), seek medical advice. Serotonin syndrome can be very serious if left untreated.

Serotonin syndrome should be confirmed by a doctor, as other conditions have similar symptoms. It's under diagnosed, as there's no single test to detect it. Doctors should be suspicious of telltale signs such as hyperreflexia, autonomic instability, and decreased platelets.

Be upfront about all medications, supplements, and substances, legal and otherwise, you've taken over the last couple of weeks. That includes when you took them, dose changes, and when your symptoms started.[3]

Alcohol

We talked previously about how alcohol, caffeine, tobacco, and cannabis can affect mental health. People taking antidepressants or other medications often ask if they can drink alcohol with their medication.

The official (or cautious) answer is that you shouldn't. Alcohol is a depressant and may worsen medication side effects. Alcohol may affect you differently when you're on the medication than before you started it. It may also change the effect of the medication. Quite frankly, the interaction between alcohol and most medications has not been studied in any great detail.

Despite this, you may plan to drink alcohol. If so, try a small amount in a safe environment. Don't drive or operate heavy machinery. Consider decreasing the amount of alcohol and limiting it to special occasions. Realize that, even then, it may counteract the effects of your medication.

Summary

- Antidepressants are complex. Careful selection, start up, monitoring, and adjustment is needed. Patient education can set expectations but is often neglected.
- Antidepressants are used for depression, anxiety, many other mental illnesses, and even a few physical illnesses. They are used very carefully, if at all, in people with bipolar disorders, as they can trigger an episode of hypomania or mania.
- Antidepressants may take weeks to work. Finding the right dose and dealing with side effects when you start them can take time and some expertise. Stopping them needs to be done gradually to prevent withdrawal.
- Choosing an antidepressant is complicated. Genetics play a role. Your symptoms are associated with different neurotransmitters, which can help. Metabolism, medication interactions, and secondary effects also factor in.

26

Other Medications

In the previous chapter, we discussed one category of psychotropic medications: antidepressants. In the process, you learned a lot about neurotransmitters, dosing, metabolism, interactions, and more. We'll try not to bombard you like that again.

But, that knowledge will be helpful in this chapter. Here, we'll cover psychotropic medication categories including sedatives and hypnotics, mood stabilizers, antipsychotics, and stimulants and related medications. As before, we'll discuss these in a general way. Details of individual medications can be found in *Appendix C*.

Sedatives and Hypnotics

Sedatives, also called anxiolytics, are medications that reduce anxiety and help you feel calm. Hypnotics help you fall asleep or stay asleep. Many medications can be used for both purposes, depending on the dose. Examples of sedatives and hypnotics include alprazolam (Xanax), diazepam (Valium), clonazepam (Klonopin, Rivotril), and zolpidem (Ambien).

You've already learned that antidepressants are used to manage many different symptoms including anxiety. In fact, serotonergic antidepressants are the psychotropic treatment of choice for most forms of ongoing anxiety. While some people are almost always anxious, others have episodes of anxiety occurring only at certain times or when faced with loss or a stressful event. In this section, we'll look at medications for such episodic anxiety. Most of these medications work quickly but aren't intended for long-term use. This is in contrast with antidepressants which take several weeks to work and can be taken long term.

The most common sedatives and hypnotics are a class of medications called *benzodiazepines* ("benzos"). Though not technically benzodiazepines, some insomnia medications such as zopiclone and zolpidem (the "z-drugs") work similarly. Note that other medications, made for entirely different purposes, can also manage anxiety-related symptoms.

Uses

Sedatives and hypnotics treat more than anxiety and insomnia. They can also decrease agitation, muscle spasms, seizures, and alcohol withdrawal.

Because many of these medications take effect very quickly, they can be used as needed[1] during stressful situations. They can also be used regularly for up to a few weeks at a time. Ongoing, daily use of sedatives and hypnotics for long periods (months or years) is controversial. More on this shortly.

How They Work

All benzodiazepines (and the z-drugs) work on the neurotransmitter GABA (gamma-aminobutyric acid). GABA is the primary inhibitory neurotransmitter. The more GABA bound to a neuron's receptors, the less likely it is to send a signal to its connected neurons. This effect is the opposite of primarily excitatory neurotransmitters such as dopamine or glutamate. When those neurotransmitters bind to a neuron's receptors, the neuron is more likely to send a signal. GABA helps to slow down and reduce signals travelling through the nervous system. It helps your body and mind calm down and relax.

Other sedatives and hypnotics use a variety of mechanisms. Some work on other neurotransmitters such as serotonin. Some blood pressure medications and antihistamines also fit into this category.

What to Expect

Medications such as benzodiazepines are much simpler to use than antidepressants. You'll feel their effects only minutes to hours after taking each pill. There's no lengthy period of adjusting to the medication or waiting weeks to see if it works. Yet, they can have side effects. If you've been on one for a while, you will need to stop it slowly to avoid withdrawal.

The most common side effects of sedatives and hypnotics are oversedation and fatigue. That's probably not surprising given they promote relaxation. They may also cause dizziness, stumbling, and problems with coordination. Until you know how they affect you, use extreme caution when you must be alert and react quickly. Driving is a good example. Higher doses are associated with more severe side effects.

Cognitively, you may experience brain fog or forgetfulness. By slowing down the nervous system, benzodiazepines can worsen depressive symptoms over time. Other changes can include an increase in anxiety, aggression, hyperactivity, irritability, agitation, or anger.

You'll likely find it harder to stop these medications the longer you've been on them and the higher the dose. You can develop a physical dependence, as with prolonged alcohol use. Withdrawal symptoms can be severe, even causing seizures. Don't stop all at once! Decreasing too fast is a widespread problem. Work with your doctor to slowly lower the dose.

>
> For people having difficulty decreasing benzodiazepines due to severe withdrawal, there are solutions. You read in the previous chapter that fluoxetine can smooth out antidepressant withdrawal. In the same way, diazepam (Valium) can reduce benzodiazepine withdrawal. It, too, remains in your system for several days. Switching to diazepam and then slowly reducing its dosage results in lighter withdrawal symptoms.[2]

Selecting a Medication

All benzodiazepines have modest differences in their effects. They vary in strength, how long they take to start working, and how long their effect lasts. Like with other medications, you may react differently than someone else.

It's important for your doctor to match the medication to your specific needs. Short-acting ones (e.g., lasting about an hour) help you fall asleep but not stay asleep. They treat panic attacks. Long-acting ones (e.g., lasting up to a day or more) are best for ongoing anxiety. You'd need several doses of a short-acting one during the day to help with ongoing anxiety, and if not taken at regular intervals, you may experience an anxiety spike or withdrawal leading up to each dose.

There are several dozen different sedatives and hypnotics. Besides benzodiazepines, many other medications also help with certain forms of anxiety. Some are even safe for long-term use. Many of these medications were created for other purposes, e.g., lowering blood pressure or reducing pain. *Appendix C* describes some of the most common ones.

Other Considerations

As mentioned, long-term daily use of benzodiazepines and similar medications is controversial. Most can be addictive. You can develop tolerance, needing a larger dose to achieve the same effect, and dependence, making them hard to stop. Using them for a short period or even occasionally over a long period does not carry the same risks.

Benzodiazepines are readily available and cause feelings of well-being and relaxation. This makes them some of the most commonly abused prescription medications. People often mix them with other substances, prescribed or otherwise, that also relax or slow body systems. These include opioid painkillers, alcohol, and illicit drugs. Combining these can be dangerous. Other medications can also compound this effect. Too much of any of these can slow your respiratory system to the point you stop breathing. You are at greater risk if you have a lung condition like asthma or sleep apnea. The opioid crisis has highlighted the dangers of accidental overdose deaths from respiratory depression.

Benzodiazepines can cause other dangers related to oversedation. These include falls and accidents while driving or operating machinery. Sedation worsens with age, making it a serious problem in seniors who are already at much higher risk of harm from falls. Long-term benzodiazepine use can also lead to memory impairment. This is again of increasing concern as people age. They increase the risk of depression and mood problems such as emotional blunting (feeling numb and unable to experience a full range of emotions).

These challenges are partly why antidepressants and other medications are the primary long-term treatments for anxiety.

Mood Stabilizers

The next medications we'll discuss are mood stabilizers. These help with bipolar disorders, illnesses consisting of both depressive episodes and hypomanic or manic (high) episodes. During a high, you may need less sleep, have racing thoughts or excess energy, or undertake risk-taking behaviours for several days. The previous chapter includes a full list of symptoms.

Mood stabilizers include lithium, valproic acid (Depakote or Epival), carbamazepine (Tegretol), and lamotrigine (Lamictal). Many other medications are used as mood stabilizers, including many antipsychotics. We'll cover these separately later in this chapter.

Uses

While antidepressants can help treat depressive episodes in bipolar disorders, their use raises the risk of hypomania or mania. Mood stabilizers help keep you from developing a mood episode, either high or low. This neutral state is known as euthymia. Treatment to keep you euthymic is called maintenance. If a mood episode develops, higher doses of mood stabilizers and other medications are briefly used to achieve remission.

Less commonly, mood stabilizers help people with unipolar depression, i.e., who have never had a hypomanic or manic episode. Some people who don't improve with antidepressants respond well to mood stabilizers.

How They Work

Let's first examine some of the biological changes associated with bipolar disorders. We know depression can result from reduced transmission of serotonin, norepinephrine, and dopamine. Too much of these, particularly of the latter two, can contribute to hypomania or mania. But other neurotransmitters are also involved during a high. Two excitatory neurotransmitters, glutamate and aspartate, act to rev up various body systems. Think of these as the reverse of GABA that you read about earlier. Finally, chemical reactions involving sodium, calcium, and potassium can put neurons into overdrive. This increases the transmission of all neurotransmitters.

Mood stabilizers work on many of these substances. Interestingly, aside from lithium, the major mood stabilizers are all anticonvulsants. Their main use is to prevent seizures in people with conditions such as epilepsy. They all affect sodium or calcium in the neuron, which changes transmission rates and reduces glutamate and aspartate. Some may also boost GABA or serotonin. The exact mechanisms by which these medications work for bipolar disorders are not fully known.

What to Expect

A bipolar disorder can be one of the more challenging illnesses to treat. The inherent mix of low and high mood states requires a complex balancing act. Finding an effective medication regime can be tricky and often takes a combination of medications.

Like antidepressants, the dosage of mood stabilizers can only be increased in small increments. Some may take weeks to have full effect. Increasing too quickly boosts the chances of having side effects. You may need lab tests before starting and more to find the right dose. Doctors often prescribe antipsychotics and benzodiazepines to manage your symptoms in the interim. Both take effect quickly.

Mood stabilizers have similar side effects to antidepressants, including gastrointestinal problems, dizziness, and headache. Weight gain and sedation can also be problematic. Your doctor should help you watch and manage these. Each medication also has rare but potentially dangerous side effects. Make sure you know what to look out for.

While withdrawal symptoms from mood stabilizers tend to be milder than with antidepressants, they do occur. Decreasing the dose gradually often helps. If you're at all prone to seizures, a sudden stop increases this risk. Also, suddenly stopping carries a high risk of developing a mood episode. This is particularly the case if you've been on the medication for a long time.

Monitoring

As with all psychotropic medications, you need to watch for specific side effects and be aware of mood changes. Mood stabilizers, except for lamotrigine, also require periodic lab monitoring.

Doses for antidepressants (and lamotrigine) are based on how well they manage your symptoms (or produce side effects). For other mood stabilizers, the level of medication in your bloodstream is critical. Blood tests check if the concentration is within a certain therapeutic level. In general, below that level, the mood stabilizer is unlikely to have much effect. Above the therapeutic level, it can be toxic.

Besides medication levels, each can potentially have side effects when used long term. Regular monitoring of weight, blood chemistry, kidneys, liver, etc. can detect problems before they become dangerous. Each medication has a protocol outlining what needs to be monitored and how often. Make sure your doctor doesn't forget this part.

Selecting a Medication

Lithium was first used to treat bipolar disorders more than 50 years ago. Options for mood stabilization have multiplied since then. While lithium is still used today, so are many other agents, alone, or in combination. The mood stabilizers listed in *Appendix C* are part of that mix, but so are various antipsychotics and sometimes antidepressants.

Your physical health may preclude the use of some medications. Your pattern of mood episodes may favour some medications as a starting point. You will likely undergo some trial and error before you find the best medication regime. For many people, no regime is ideal, and they struggle with a balancing act between highs, lows, and side effects. Keep track of your symptoms and medication changes. This can prevent your doctor from changing your medication based solely on how you're feeling the day of your appointment.

Antipsychotics

When a doctor suggests you take an antipsychotic, you may question why you require the same hardcore medication used for a severe illness such as schizophrenia. You're not alone. In truth, doctors use antipsychotics even when psychosis isn't an issue. They treat depression, anxiety, bipolar disorders, PTSD, OCD, and some personality disorders.

Doctors use antipsychotics for mild to moderate mental illness differently than for severe illness. Doses tend to be much smaller. High doses are used rarely and for short periods, if at all. Examples of antipsychotics include quetiapine (Seroquel), risperidone (Risperdal), and olanzapine (Zyprexa).

Uses

Antipsychotics operate primarily on dopamine. Some also affect norepinephrine and serotonin. But they do so via a wider variety of mechanisms than antidepressants. This makes them uniquely capable of being added to antidepressants or other medications. They can treat problems that the "main" medication didn't fully correct. Let's look at a few uses.

- *Acute episodes.* Antipsychotics are often used to quickly control symptoms of an acute mood episode. They take effect within days, and their dose doesn't need to be slowly increased over weeks. Once you are no longer in crisis, they can be decreased or stopped altogether.

- *Transitional agents.* Antidepressants and mood stabilizers take weeks before they take full effect. Antipsychotics can manage your most bothersome symptoms until then. Their purpose here is similar to using benzodiazepines to manage anxiety in the short term.

- *Augmenting agents.* Interestingly, low doses of some antipsychotics can improve the effectiveness of antidepressants. Say your antidepressant helped you feel 80-90% better. However, you can't increase the dose further. Maybe you're at the maximum or have too many side effects. Adding a small dose of an antipsychotic may give it enough of a boost to help you feel 100% well.

- *Symptom management.* Your antidepressant or mood stabilizer may have helped with most of your symptoms. Antipsychotics can target symptoms that your main psychotropic medication isn't resolving. For example, quetiapine can help with sleep and nightmares, while risperidone can help with racing thoughts or anger. Unlike benzodiazepines which are addictive, antipsychotics may be better for long-term use.

Some people with mood problems have tried every antidepressant and mood stabilizer in the book. Even so, they can't find one (or a combination) that they can both tolerate and that treats their symptoms. An antipsychotic may fit the bill when other medications haven't worked.

How They Work

Antipsychotics can affect several neurotransmitters. All reduce dopamine transmission by blocking one type of dopamine receptor (D2). The second-generation or atypical antipsychotics also block one type of serotonin receptor (5HT2A). Some medications increase or decrease the transmission of other neurotransmitters and receptors.

Best Practices

While antipsychotics are a mainstay for treating many symptoms of mental illness, you need to proceed with caution.

Antipsychotics have side effects, especially when used long term. Weight gain is more common and more pronounced than with some antidepressants. Other risks include poor blood sugar control (which can lead to diabetes), increased cholesterol, movement disorders (tics or tremors), hormone changes, cardiac rhythm changes, and drowsiness. Remember that just because these can happen, it does not mean they will.

Other than for acute mood states, they're probably not the first tool to reach for. Still, based on your symptoms and response to other medications, adding an antipsychotic to your regime may be the best choice. Before starting, most people should have baseline measurements done (e.g., weight, abdominal circumference, ECG, glucose, lipids, liver, kidneys). Your current health may also be a factor. Ongoing monitoring, typically not long after starting and then every 6 to 12 months, should pick up any changes. The risks to your overall health, the benefits of the medication, and ways to minimize side effects should be considered.

Stimulants and Related Medications

The final class of psychotropic medications we'll look at are stimulants, along with some related non-stimulant medications. They are used to treat Attention-Deficit Hyperactivity Disorder (ADHD). Examples include amphetamine (Adderall), methylphenidate (Ritalin), and atomoxetine (Strattera).

How They Work

Stimulants boost transmission of dopamine (primarily) and norepinephrine. That results in increased attention, focus, and cognitive skills.

Broadly, there are two main types of stimulant medications. The first type derives from the stimulant amphetamine and includes Dexedrine, Adderall, and Vyvanse. The other type derives from the stimulant methylphenidate. It includes Ritalin, Concerta, and Biphentin/Aptensio. Most people find that one type or the other works better.

Otherwise, medications differ depending on how long their effects last and how they are released into your system. Some deliver a sizeable hit within the first hour that declines with time. Others release medication more equally over eight hours, so their effect stays constant.

Other Considerations

Stimulants also help with some symptoms of depression such as poor concentration and fatigue. They do, however, tend to worsen anxiety.

Though not a concern when used as prescribed, stimulants are often abused and can be addictive. Some people take large doses or crush some extended-release pills to receive a massive hit right away. The result is similar to taking cocaine, which also delivers a sudden dopamine boost. Sometimes they are mixed with other medications. People without ADHD obtain them to use as cognitive enhancers. Their use by university students during exam preparation is widespread.

There are non-stimulant treatments for ADHD which have less potential for abuse. Atomoxetine (Strattera) helps with many ADHD symptoms. It works on norepinephrine rather than dopamine. Another non-stimulant option is extended-release guanfacine (Intuniv), which also affects norepinephrine. Both can cause hypomania or mania if you are at risk.

All these medications can interact with other medications and illicit drugs. They can increase blood pressure, decrease weight, change heart rhythms, affect hormones, and cause glaucoma. Take them only under medical supervision.

Other

We've discussed antidepressants, benzodiazepines, mood stabilizers, antipsychotics, and stimulants and related medications. These are the main classes of psychotropic medications used today.

Sometimes, medications made for entirely different uses can help with psychiatric symptoms. You already read that many anticonvulsants work as mood stabilizers. Some blood pressure medications (e.g., propranolol, prazosin) can reduce nightmares. Some antihistamines (e.g., hydroxyzine) work as well as benzodiazepines for anxiety or sleep, with less risk of addiction or dependence. There are many other examples.

Different medications are used to deal with the side effects of psychotropic medications. We'll discuss those in the next chapter.

> *Summary*
>
> - Sedatives and hypnotics help with anxiety and sleep. The majority are benzodiazepines. They can cause tolerance, dependence, oversedation, and cognitive problems if used long term.
>
> - Mood stabilizers prevent both depressive and hypomanic or manic episodes. They are used to treat bipolar disorders but also unipolar depression. Some of them need periodic monitoring to avoid long-term health problems.
>
> - Antipsychotics in high doses help with psychotic illnesses. In lower doses, they can be used for other illnesses. They can help in the short term before an antidepressant starts working. They can boost the effectiveness of antidepressants or help long term with symptoms such as insomnia, anger, or rumination.
>
> - Stimulants help with attention, focus, and other cognitive skills associated with ADHD. They can help treat some symptoms in other illnesses such as depression.

27

Medication Side Effects

In this chapter, we'll first summarize the information about side effects we've already mentioned. We'll then review key questions you should ask yourself if you think you may be experiencing a medication side effect. Finally, we'll describe how to manage those which are most common.

When deciding if a medication should remain in your living treatment plan, you need to consider its effectiveness, its side effects, and treatment alternatives. Giving up on a medication because of a mild side effect may keep you away from an effective treatment. At the same time, don't accept a bothersome side effect without at least discussing it with your doctor. You may be suffering needlessly.

Our key message is this: treatment is a balancing act, so talk to your doctor about your medication side effects.

General Strategies

Over the last few chapters, you've already learned a few important things about side effects:

- Just because a medication may cause a side effect does not mean you will have that side effect. A common side effect is one that affects fewer than 1 in 10 people taking a medication and maybe as few as 1 in 100. Those are pretty good odds.
- Side effects vary in severity, from barely there, to noticeable, to slightly annoying, to completely debilitating. The severity of a side effect should influence what action you take, if any.

- Most side effects occur within the first few days of starting a medication or when changing the dose. Most decline over several days to a couple of weeks. They may disappear entirely given enough time.
- Your expectations affect how you experience side effects. If you anticipate a terrible ordeal, you are more likely to find side effects more intense or bothersome. Side effects can be caused by anxiety, instead of the medication.[1]
- Similar medications can have vastly different side effect profiles.

Will you experience a medication's side effect, and if so, how bad will it be? Unfortunately, science hasn't provided a reliable way to answer these questions yet. Population-wide statistics remain your best bet. Here's how to interpret words such as "common" and "rare":

- very common: experienced by more than 10% of people taking the medication;
- common: between 1%–10%;
- uncommon: between 0.1%–1%;
- rare: between 0.01%–0.1%;
- very rare: fewer than 0.01%.

The consumer website drugs.com identifies the frequency of side effects for most medications.

We've discussed these approaches to managing side effects:

- *Wait. Wait some more. Then wait some more.* There may be no point dealing with something that will disappear over time.
- *Go lower and slower.* If you have side effects when increasing the medication dose, increase the dose by a smaller amount and at a slower rate. This also applies if you have withdrawal when decreasing the dose. The standard dosing schedules are too aggressive for many people. The next chapter discusses options, such as splitting pills or compounding, if smaller doses aren't commercially available.
- *Change how you take the medication.* Would taking it at a different time of day help? If it causes fatigue, take it in the evening. Does taking it with or without food make a difference? What about splitting one large dose into two smaller ones taken at two separate times?
- *Does a slightly lower dose reduce side effects?* If so, how much does that worsen symptoms? Could boosting or augmenting the lower dose

with another medication help? Consider non-medication treatments that could reduce how much medication you need, e.g., diet, sleep, exercise, and therapy.

- *Can you work around the side effects?* In other words, are there things you can do to avoid or minimize them? You might add another medication or natural supplement to treat the side effect. Or are there behaviour changes that could help? For example, improving your sleep hygiene can reduce the impact of medication-induced insomnia.
- *Try another medication?* Weigh the cost of the side effect, the benefit from the medication, the time needed to slowly stop the current medication, and the risk involved with another medication. If the side effect is greatly impacting your life and is tough to work around, trying another medication is probably the right answer.

Get Help or Wait?

Usually, waiting to see if a side effect will resolve on its own is the right thing to do. But that's not always the case. Some things, typically quite rare, need to be dealt with right away. These include a severe allergic reaction or passing out from a large drop in blood pressure.

Don't toss the information leaflet the pharmacist gives you when you pick up your medication. It tells you what to do if you encounter specific side effects. You may need to immediately stop it, seek medical attention, or call your doctor or pharmacist for advice. If you did throw away the information, you can find patient medication handouts on consumer websites such as drugs.com or rxlist.com.

Some medications have side effects which aren't urgent but can be serious if not dealt with. For example, the anticonvulsants lamotrigine or carbamazepine can cause a rash. Left untreated, some rashes could develop into Stevens-Johnson Syndrome, which can sometimes be fatal over time. When starting these medications, your doctor or pharmacist will usually tell you what to watch for and what to do if a rash appears.

Waiting is the right approach when dealing with most side effects. If in doubt, ask your pharmacist or doctor.[2] When you describe your side effects, try to be as specific as possible.

Sexual Dysfunction

Some side effects concern people more than others and can deter them from starting a medication. Sexual side effects are high on that list. They are also a frequently given reason that medications are stopped prematurely.

Sexual side effects usually fall into one or more of three categories. The first is reduced sexual desire or libido. The second is a decrease in arousal. Men have difficulty developing or maintaining an erection. Women experience inadequate lubrication and swelling of their genitals. The third is greater delay or difficulty reaching orgasm or inability to orgasm.

Much of the general advice applies to sexual dysfunction. Changes in dose and timing can help, as can increasing exercise and decreasing alcohol use. A similar medication may not cause you problems, even if it also carries a risk of sexual side effects. Sexual problems can also be caused by other stressors or be symptoms of a mental or physical illness needing further treatment. If sexual side effects occur, they may diminish over time. Unfortunately, this is less likely than with side effects such as nausea or headache.

Beyond the general approaches to side effects, there are several options to consider.[3] Each has benefits and risks that depend on your situation and physical health. Discuss these with a family doctor or psychiatrist who knows all aspects of your health:

- The antidepressant bupropion (Wellbutrin) is widely used to reduce or counteract the full range of sexual side effects of other medications. It can, however, increase anxiety, irritability, and, for those with a bipolar disorder, rarely precipitate a hypomanic or manic episode.

- For men, medications such as sildenafil (Viagra) and tadalafil (Cialis) can usually resolve erectile problems. While there have been suggestions that these medications may have some benefit for women, evidence either supporting or refuting this is limited.

- Problematic medications can be temporarily decreased or stopped for a few days during so-called *medication holidays*. These may temporarily reduce sexual side effects but only work for medications with a moderate half-life. They don't work for medications such as fluoxetine (Prozac) that stay in your system for many weeks after you stop it. They also may not work with medications such as venlafaxine (Effexor) or paroxetine (Paxil) which leave your system quickly when stopped and thereby cause severe withdrawal. Medication holidays increase the risk of your mental health deteriorating or premature discontinuation of your medication altogether.

- Several other medications reduce sexual side effects when taken before sex. Their effectiveness and clinical evidence vary. These include the antihistamine cyproheptadine, the anxiolytic buspirone (Buspar), the alpha-adrenergic blocker yohimbine, the antiparkinsonian amantadine, and stimulant medications for ADHD.
- A few natural supplements have also been used to reduce the impact of sexual side effects. What limited clinical evidence is available is mainly in the form of case reports. Common supplements include natural yohimbine extracts, maca root, ginkgo biloba, and saffron. Acupuncture has some limited evidence for use in this context.

Curious why these various solutions work or why so many psychotropic medications can cause sexual side effects? Neurotransmitters! Sexual function is complicated and depends on the levels of multiple neurotransmitters and hormones. Here are some of the main ones:

- Libido relies on adequate levels of dopamine, testosterone, and estrogen, among others. It can drop not only with low levels of these but also high levels of other substances such as prolactin. Prolactin can increase with psychotropic use.
- Arousal relies on dopamine and norepinephrine, as well as two other neurotransmitters, acetylcholine and nitric oxide.
- The ability to orgasm is improved with increased levels of norepinephrine but can be impaired by too much serotonin. SSRIs increase the level of serotonin in your genitals, causing a decrease in function.

Not surprisingly, the various treatments noted above rely on these mechanisms. Bupropion boosts norepinephrine and dopamine. Erectile dysfunction medications boost nitric oxide. Buspirone and cyproheptadine work on two different serotonin receptors. Yohimbine indirectly boosts norepinephrine. Finally, amantadine and various stimulants boost dopamine.

Weight Gain

Possible weight gain is a concern with many medications, psychotropic medications among them. It's most common with antipsychotic and some mood stabilizing medications. Some people feel severe anguish at the thought of taking any medication that may cause weight gain. If this is a concern, have a frank conversation with your doctor up front. Emphasize the importance of addressing any weight gain. As always, even though weight gain can occur, it doesn't mean it will. It's worth noting that weight gain can be a symptom of depression and other mental illnesses. Many people also put on weight from binge eating to cope with their distress.

Weight gain can lead to many health conditions, including cardiovascular disease and diabetes. Signs to watch for include high blood pressure, high blood glucose levels, excess fat in the abdominal area, and abnormalities in cholesterol and triglycerides. Baseline measurements should be taken before starting a medication with a high potential for weight gain. Periodic measurement while you're taking the medication should catch any changes early. They then can be addressed before they turn into serious health issues.

One option to deal with weight gain is switching to another medication. That, of course, carries its own challenges. As with weight gain from other causes, behavioural modification, such as changes in diet, exercise, and education around nutrition is preferred. Some forms of cognitive behavioural therapy and mindfulness are also effective.

> Though not the preferred choice, medications may play a role. Your doctor may suggest these to help control your blood sugar (e.g., metformin) or cholesterol (e.g., a statin). There are a few prescription anti-obesity medications that are currently approved. Be aware that many past anti-obesity medications were pulled from the market due in part to psychiatric issues. Caution is therefore warranted. Similarly, be very careful with over-the-counter weight loss medications and supplements. Many of these are stimulants that can worsen some psychiatric issues and interact with psychotropic medications. The anticonvulsant topiramate is sometimes used off-label, i.e. unofficially, to help with weight loss. It does have mood stabilizing properties but can cause brain fog.

Sleep Problems

Problems falling or staying asleep are both symptoms of some mental illnesses. They are also side effects of some psychotropic medications. Unfortunately, sleep issues can worsen your mental health. But, a variety of approaches can help.[4] Adjusting when you take a medication may be enough. For instance, take a more stimulating medication earlier in the day.

Medications or supplements can be a short-term solution. Over-the-counter products such as antihistamines and short-acting or long-acting melatonin are commonly helpful. Your doctor might prescribe a benzodiazepine or a z-drug such as zolpidem or zopiclone. These can be problematic when used long term. Sedating antidepressants are frequently prescribed along with other medications to help with sleep. Trazodone, doxepin, and mirtazapine are the most common of these. The older antihistamine hydroxyzine is also used. Both the blood pressure medication prazosin and the antipsychotic quetiapine can reduce nightmares. These add-on medications may help you but have their own side effects.

If you have long-term sleep issues, however, prescription and over-the-counter medications and supplements are usually not the answer. The best solution is improving your *sleep hygiene*. This collection of habits and practices was described in the *Lifestyle Factors* chapter. Another option is a specific form of cognitive behavioural therapy that has been proven to help with insomnia. If insomnia or fatigue remains problematic, ask your doctor if you need tests for sleep apnea or another sleep disorder.

Anticholinergic Symptoms

One group of symptoms is caused by a decrease in the neurotransmitter acetylcholine, a common effect of many medications, including some psychotropics. These symptoms are therefore termed *anticholinergic* side effects.[5]

These include dry mouth, constipation, urinary retention, bowel obstruction, dilated pupils, blurred vision, palpitations, decreased sweating, impaired concentration, brain fog, decreased attention, memory impairment, sedation, and dizziness.

Because so many medications have anticholinergic side effects, family doctors have a lot of experience with managing them. After reviewing your medication list, they can adjust the doses or change them altogether. There are also some medications, e.g., bethanechol, which have a cholinergic effect, increasing acetylcholine and thereby reducing these side effects. Deficiencies of the nutrient choline are also common.[6] You may need to address this with diet changes or supplements.

Keep in mind that many anticholinergic symptoms are relatively nonspecific and have multiple other possible causes.

Anticholinergic medications can be deliberately added to counteract other medication side effects. For example, many medications can increase sweating. Anticholinergic medications such as benztropine (Cogentin) can help.

Cognitive Problems

Cognitive side effects include changes in memory, attention, concentration, problem-solving, multitasking, processing speed, and reaction time. These can result from the anticholinergic effects of medications. They also occur with benzodiazepines, antipsychotics, and some anticonvulsants. Medications aren't always the cause of these problems. They can be due to underlying illnesses such as depression or ADHD. Alcohol or substance use can contribute. So can poor sleep, a lack of exercise, or many dietary deficiencies. Identifying and addressing any of these factors is usually the first step.

After that, identifying and switching or reducing doses of anticholinergic medications such as paroxetine (Paxil), some tricyclic antidepressants, and some antipsychotics is often recommended. Adding other medications may help address cognitive problems in people with depression or anxiety. Most common are psychostimulants. These include amphetamine, methylphenidate, or modafinil. Other medications that increase dopamine, such as some for Parkinson's disease, or cholinesterase inhibitors, which help cognitive symptoms in Alzheimer's patients, have been investigated, but trials have been mostly inconclusive.

Twitching and Restlessness

A variety of different side effects related to agitation, restlessness, and muscle twitching can occur. When they happen, they are often benign, but they can become annoying if frequent or severe.

Akathisia is a feeling of inner restlessness. It can make it difficult to sit still. This leads you to fidget, rock back and forth, and repeatedly cross and uncross your legs. Many people feel stressed or irritable and describe wanting to climb out of their skin. Beta blockers such as propranolol (Inderal) are usually the first medications prescribed. Some Parkinson's medications can also be used. Benzodiazepines such as lorazepam (Ativan) can help, but for short-term use only.

Restless legs often respond well to dopamine agonists such as pramipexole (Mirapex), gabapentin, or pregabalin (Lyrica). Low iron (ferritin < 50) can be a contributing factor and must be treated.

Involuntary muscle twitches are usually benign. They can be worsened by dehydration, low magnesium, or low calcium. If intrusive, medications such as propranolol or clonazepam are often used.

A persistent tremor should be evaluated by a doctor. It can be perfectly harmless. It can be due to many physical conditions, some mild, and some serious. It may be an indication of medication toxicity.

Others

Over-the-counter treatments are readily available for many side effects, at least in the short term:

- Headaches and other pain may be relieved with a wide range of over-the-counter medications, e.g., Tylenol, Advil.

- For dry mouth, try chewing sugarless gum, or using a product such as Biotene.

- Diarrhea or constipation may respond to diet changes (e.g., adding fibre), or medications such as bismuth subsalicylate (Pepto-Bismol), loperamide (Imodium), or PEG 3350 (Miralax). Be aware that some of these products affect how you absorb medication; check with your pharmacist.

- For nausea, try ginger products or bismuth subsalicylate. Dimenhydrinate (Gravol/Dramamine) has a strong anticholinergic effect, and so may or may not be advised.

Prescription medications are also available for the above concerns. For example, both ondansetron (Zofran) and mirtazapine (Remeron) affect the serotonin receptors that cause most psychotropic-induced nausea. If over-the-counter preparations aren't sufficient, ask your doctor.

> ### *Summary*
>
> - Side effects can occur with all medications but can be managed. You should know which ones need to be dealt with immediately and which can wait. Your expectations and anxiety can worsen side effects.
>
> - Most side effects from psychotropic medications occur when starting or increasing the dose and often go away on their own over a few days or weeks. Waiting is often the right approach.
>
> - Most side effects can be resolved by decreasing the medication dose, changing when you take the medication, or using other treatments to address the side effect. Abandoning a medication immediately due to a side effect may be a lost opportunity.
>
> - There are specific strategies that can help manage side effects including sexual dysfunction, weight gain, and sleep problems.

28

Evolving Your Medication Regime

In the previous few chapters, we've described how psychotropic medications work, how they can help, and why they are used. We've highlighted essential information about the major classes of medications and explained how to manage side effects.

You may have a pretty good idea which medications will meet your needs. You may have even talked with your doctor and started taking one. Every once in a while, the initial dose of the first medication you try will be all you need to thoroughly treat your symptoms without causing side effects. In mental health, that is most definitely the exception and not the rule, but it can happen.

Assuming you didn't 100% succeed on your first try, you should work with your doctor to make changes. You'll consider questions such as these:

- Should you increase the dose?
- If so, by how much?
- How long should you wait before increasing?
- Should you try something else?
- Is the new medication in addition to or replacing what you're taking?
- How do you decrease a medication that isn't working?
- If you have side effects, what then?

Why So Difficult?

Because everyone reacts differently to mental health medications, there are no universal answers to these questions. It will take trial and error to find the right combination of medication(s) and dose(s) for you.

We've emphasized the importance of giving a medication a proper trial. You don't want to reject a medication that actually could help. Unfortunately, this happens far too often. A proper medication trial requires both you and your doctor to have realistic expectations about what effects you hope to see and when you hope to see them. What you see and when may be very different from others on the same medication.

Common missteps with medication trials include these:

- You don't wait long enough to see an effect.
- You stop at the initial dose, even if it's below the target dose (the dose that helps most people who benefit from the medication).
- You immediately stop when you first experience any uncomfortable side effect.
- You and your doctor make incorrect assumptions. For example, your doctor assumes you took your medication as and when prescribed. Instead, you took less and started later than planned.
- You try a standard dose that is too high (or increases too fast) for you to tolerate, but don't try again lower and slower.
- You discount other health problems or life stressors and blame how you feel entirely on the medication.

It's easy to end a promising trial prematurely, particularly if your doctor doesn't prescribe a medication often or if they don't know you well.

Document the Process

While you and your doctor work to find the right medication regime, document the process. Use your living treatment plan to keep track:

- Understand why you're trying each medication, i.e., what problem will this medication hopefully solve? How does it fit into the big picture?
- Describe what each step of the trial looks like. What are the doses? How long do you need to wait?
- Measure the extent to which the medication helps or not.

As you begin trying anything new, add it to your living treatment plan. Every time you make a change, e.g., start a medication or increase the dose, make a note. If what you tried doesn't work, whether the medication doesn't help or you can't tolerate it, record it as an unsuccessful treatment. Write down why it didn't work.

Ideally, you should make one change at a time. But as we said, sometimes it makes sense to try several things at once. Starting several medications at once is not common, but it happens. Adjusting doses of several medications is more common.

Expectations and Evaluation

At each new step, find out what to expect. Ask your doctor what effect you could see and how long it might take. This determines how long to spend on a given step.

You'll recall that antidepressants require several weeks before they take full effect. You need to increase them slowly, and you may not even expect any improvement at lower doses. These first steps help you adjust to and tolerate the medication. Evaluating the benefits will happen later.

When making any medication change, expect some side effects. Most side effects happen when first starting a medication or changing its dose. Many go away quickly, often in days, sometimes weeks. Most are not dangerous, though they may be uncomfortable or annoying.

When you evaluate a medication change, ask yourself if other factors played a part. Recent events, good or bad, can affect your mood and overall mental health. The last thing you want is to make medication changes based on a quick snapshot of how you feel at your doctor's appointment. Consider how you've been feeling over several days or weeks and if any events or stressors influenced your mood. Plan what you want to tell your doctor ahead of the appointment. Ask family and friends for their input.

Adjustments

At each appointment, you'll evaluate how well your medication is working and consult your treatment plan. Then you and your doctor will figure out the next step. The next step may include not making any change at all. Instead, you may decide to wait a bit longer on your current medication regime. In effect, you're extending the timeframe of the current step.

You may decide to keep your medication as-is for the long term. Your next step then is to do nothing. No more tweaks, no more trials. Your current medication regime has treated your symptoms and helped you meet your goals. In other words, it worked!

Another reason to not make a change is that the medication partly helped, and you figure that's good enough for now. It's okay to adjust your goals. Perhaps you don't want to make any more changes right now, but you'll come back to it later. Sometimes you just need a break from always feeling like a patient. But long term, you should aim for full remission of your symptoms.

Then, of course, there are the changes you can make to your medications to see what effect they will have: changing the dose, adding another medication, or discontinuing the medication.

Change Dosage

Increasing or decreasing the dose of a medication is the most common type of change you'll make. You and your doctor may decide to increase your dose if you've tolerated your current dose, notice some benefit, but think that a higher dose may give a better result.

Similarly, you may decrease your dose if the higher dose you tried didn't work. Maybe you had no added benefit, in which case why take more medication when less will do? Maybe a side effect became worse, or you couldn't tolerate the increase. Perhaps the higher dose worsened your initial mental health symptoms. For example, venlafaxine helps anxiety at low doses because it affects serotonin. As you increase the dose, it also boosts norepinephrine and dopamine, which may increase anxiety.

Sometimes psychotropic medications are increased too quickly. By making slower increases, your body has time to get used to the medication. If you are sensitive to medications, consider starting at half the typical starting dose and waiting twice as long between dose increases.

Sometimes the smallest size pill available is the usual starting dose. If so, ask your doctor or pharmacist if it can be split, which some medications can. Others, however, should never be divided. Splitting many extended-release pills will cause you to absorb a large amount of medication at once, instead of over time as intended. If they can be split, divide tablets with an X-acto knife or similar precision blade, or a dedicated pill splitter. Many capsules can be opened, and their contents divided.

> For example, the smallest dose of duloxetine (Cymbalta) in Canada is 30 mg. Two 15-mg capsules can be made by twisting open a 30-mg capsule, dividing the enteric-coated pellets inside between the halves, and then sealing each half with a bit of bread or soft cheese.
>
> Other tricks may be available. Again with duloxetine, half the pellets can be added to applesauce, and the other half saved in the original capsule. What works really depends on the medication. Don't try to put duloxetine in chocolate pudding, even though this works for many other medications.[1]

You can also enlist the help of a compounding pharmacy to produce any dose of most medications. Because this takes time and manpower, these are unfortunately more expensive than standard commercial doses.

Medication changes might also involve keeping the total dosage the same but changing when you take it. If a medication is too sedating when taken in the morning, try taking it in the evening instead. Or, if a particular dose taken once a day causes a bad side effect, splitting the dose and taking it at two different times might help. Sometimes even changing to the same medication made by a different company may make a difference. Some people react to the colourings, fillers, and other non-medicinal ingredients. Compounding pharmacies can come in handy here, too.

Add Another Medication

You could add a new medication to what you're already taking. It may boost or augment the effectiveness of your existing medication, as when adding low doses of antipsychotics to antidepressants. Alternatively, it may treat other symptoms or manage side effects of your current medications. Adding bupropion to an SSRI may increase energy or reduce sexual side effects.

Keep track of why you're trying to add another medication. That's where your living treatment plan shines. You don't want to add a second medication to treat the side effects of one that isn't providing any benefit.

> Adding new medications is something that doctors tend to be very good at doing. Stopping medications—not so much. Many hesitate to stop a treatment prescribed by another doctor, especially if they don't know why it was started in the first place. Understanding your medications and why you're taking them helps avoid this problem. Your living treatment plan should explain the "why" of every medication to any doctor you see.
>
> Many people are prescribed too many medications, some treating side effects of medications they're no longer using. Overprescribing is a real problem, particularly affecting seniors.
>
> Sadly, it's not unusual to see people on a crazy cocktail of medications, half of which are working at cross purposes. They probably cause more side effects than actual benefits. We've seen people taking four different benzodiazepines, three antidepressants, two mood stabilizers, an antipsychotic, a stimulant, and then other medications to treat side effects, e.g., pain killers for headaches and anti-nausea meds. That medication regime did not appear overnight. Fixing it is time-consuming and difficult.

Discontinue

Stopping a medication is another action you and your doctor might decide to take. You may find the medication isn't helpful or the side effects are more annoying or intolerable than you expected. Maybe you've been on the medication for a long time and want to see if you can get by without it. Occasionally, medications simply stop working after a few years, usually referred to as *pooping out.*

If you stop your medications as soon as you no longer have any symptoms, your symptoms are likely to return. As we mentioned in the *Antidepressants* chapter, guidelines recommend how long you should continue a medication to minimize the chance of relapse.

Most medications need to be gradually reduced to prevent significant withdrawal symptoms. Again, everyone reacts differently.

If you plan to stop your current medication and try another, your doctor might ask you to slowly add the new one as you're reducing the old one. You can *cross-taper* only some pairs of medications this way. It can both save time and minimize withdrawal as it keeps a roughly even amount of medication in your system.

Special Situations

There are several special situations such as overseas travel, surgery, and pregnancy, that may require changes to your psychotropic medication regime. A trip to your prescribing doctor is usually advisable. In this section, we'll quickly note some of the most common situations that arise, and then introduce some strategies to deal with them.

Pregnancy

Whether to continue your psychotropic medications during pregnancy can be a difficult choice. Can they pose a risk to fetal growth and development? Can they cause pre-term delivery or birth defects? While we can't begin to do justice to this issue here, consider the following:

- Up to 3% of healthy mothers, doing everything right and not taking any medications, can have a child with a congenital defect. Statistics on individual defects are also available.[2]
- Some psychotropic medications can increase these risks. Some are associated with one or more specific defects. Other medications have been well studied, and no risks to the fetus or related to the pregnancy itself have been found. Still others have not been studied much so there's less known about their risks.

- Consider the total size of the risk, not just how much a medication increases it. A three times greater risk for a defect that otherwise is present in 1 of every 5,000 births (0.06% versus 0.02%) may or may not be important to you. Put that into context of other risks. For example, the effect of smoking on low birth weight is 9.1% versus 4.5% for non-smokers.[3] The risk may be (only) two times greater but compare the actual size of the risk.
- There are ways to decrease some risks. For instance, some mood stabilizers increase the risk of neural tube defects. Folic acid supplements can decrease this risk.
- Untreated mental illnesses can themselves significantly raise the risk of negative birth outcomes including premature birth and low birth weight. Pregnancy complications and increased emotional and developmental problems in children are also increased. Untreated mental illness is associated with poorer nutrition, riskier behaviours, and decreased compliance with prenatal care recommendations.

There is no risk-free pregnancy. You can't control everything. Your challenge is to find the right balance. The odds of most risks are still very small. With these considerations in mind, we recommend the following:

- Pregnancies should be planned. Some congenital defects appear in the initial weeks of pregnancy. Planning allows you to work with your doctor to change any medications ahead of time.
- If you become pregnant, do not suddenly stop taking medications. This can cause severe physical and psychological withdrawal and a relapse of your illness. This, in turn, raises risks to you and the fetus.[4]
- Seek advice from reputable organizations that provide information on pregnancy, e.g., OTIS.[5] They can help you understand the risks associated with your illness as well as medications and natural substances you take. Review what you have learned with your doctor.
- Be aware of your risk of becoming unwell in the postpartum period. Depression and psychosis are common. Make plans so that any problems are caught early.
- If you plan to breastfeed, there is good information available through OTIS about which medications cross into breast milk, which do not, and how this affects infants.

Hormonal Changes

Your mental health is affected by hormonal changes. Significant changes occur during puberty, during pregnancy, in the postnatal period, and during perimenopause. Hormonal changes are part of the regular menstrual cycle. Some illnesses cause hormonal changes, and many medications are either hormones themselves or affect hormone levels. Some intrauterine devices (IUDs) release hormones that negatively affect mood in a small proportion of women.

Be mindful of your mental health during times when hormone changes occur. Watch your ongoing symptoms closely and look out for any new ones. If you notice changes, be proactive and address them with your treatment team. Make sure they know about your hormonal changes. Your medications may need adjustments.

Many women who experience significant physical and mental premenstrual symptoms benefit from the addition of an SSRI. The symptoms include mood swings, marked irritability or anger, hopelessness, self-criticism, feeling overwhelmed, tension or anxiety, decreased interest and concentration, fatigue, and changes in sleep patterns and appetite. Strategies to manage this differ. SSRIs can be used either daily or only during part of the menstrual cycle. They may be started during the luteal phase (typically 10-14 days before menstruation) or only in the latter portion of that phase, coinciding with the onset of symptoms. If not used continually, they are usually discontinued at or just after the start of menstruation. Medication choice and dosage varies. As always, be careful with SSRIs if you have a bipolar disorder.

Overseas Travel

Overseas air travel can be challenging when you take psychotropic medications. Here are some things to consider before you fly:

- To minimize mental health symptoms, make sure you have adequate sleep, especially when taking long overnight flights. Ask your doctor if a temporary sleep aid would help.
- Plan ahead so you know when you will take your medications, factoring in time zone changes. Depending on the length of your trip, you might adhere to either your home or destination time zone or plan a short transition at either end.
- Research your destination ahead of time. Some countries require letters from your doctor describing what medications you take for what condition. Some may prohibit or tightly restrict certain medications, including stimulants, opioids, or benzodiazepines.
- It may not be easy or possible to obtain replacement prescriptions abroad. Keep your medications close when travelling, not in checked

luggage. If two people are travelling, consider splitting the medication between you. Bring a few extras days' worth in case of travel delays.
- Always bring your medications in their original bottles. Your pharmacy can give you properly labelled small bottles sized for your trip.

Hospitalization or Surgery

If you will be having surgery, other medical procedures, or are being admitted to hospital, make sure your entire treatment team knows what medications you're taking. Speak with the doctor who will be taking care of you in the hospital, the doctor at the pre-admission clinic, and the doctor who prescribed your medications. Find out if you will need to stop any medications or alter your schedule. This could result in significant withdrawal symptoms. Find out if the medications you are taking are available on the hospital formulary (i.e., are they stocked, or should you bring them yourself?). Planning is key.

Summary

- Finding the right medication regime to optimally address your symptoms can be challenging. Many common mistakes cause people to give up on promising medications too early.
- Carefully document all your medication changes. Be aware of how long it should take before you notice an effect. Monitor your side effects.
- Increasing or decreasing doses can be tricky for some people sensitive to medications, though workarounds are available. Adding another medication may be a better option than increasing the dose of a current one. Equally, reducing or stopping a current medication may lead you to a better option.
- Special situations such as pregnancy, travel, and surgery can sometimes mean changes to a stable medication regime. Take the time to find out what, if any, changes may be needed, and plan to make them in a controlled manner.

29

Looking Ahead

We wrote this book to help you improve your mental health in the face of what can be a bewildering, flawed, and, at times, heartless mental health system. We showed you what mental illness is all about and why good care is so difficult to find. You learned to navigate the system and improve your mental health by working collaboratively with mental health professionals. You saw how your skills and time complement what they can offer. Finally, you saw how the many treatments and interventions for mental illness fit together, what they have in common, how they differ, and how to best choose and use them.

In a moment, we'll turn our eyes to the not-too-distant future. But first, these words of advice.

Started Yet?

Are you the type who reads a self-help book cover-to-cover before starting to apply what you've learned? You have too many things buzzing through your mind, have lost track of many others, and are probably more than a bit overwhelmed. If that's the case, now is a perfect time to take stock of your current situation and take your first steps forward.

1. Start by collecting the basic tools of the trade (see the *Get Prepared* chapter). At the very least, pick one place where you can gather all your mental health information.
2. Review the *Describing Your Symptoms* chapter. Try to concisely describe what aspects of your mental health are causing you the most distress and are interfering with your life. You may want to review this with a friend or family member.

3. If you've tried some lifestyle changes, supplements, prescription medications, or therapy, write them down. Did they help, and, if so, how much?

4. Optionally, skim the typical questions in the *Mental Health Interviews* chapter. Jot down answers to those questions that particularly resonate.

5. Make an appointment with your family doctor (or, find a nearby walk-in clinic) to start the process. Don't expect an answer at your first appointment. For some tips, see the *Working With Your Family Doctor* chapter.

6. Afterwards, begin to sketch out what will evolve into your living treatment plan (see the *Your Living Treatment Plan* chapter).

Trends to Watch

We've described the benefits of being actively involved in your care. What will mental health care look like in a few years? We can make some predictions based on current trends. Will the skills you've learned here help you in the future? They may be even more important.

New Tests and Treatments

There's always something new around the corner. Genetic testing, as well as more advanced imaging, is in its early days. While you can still expect incremental changes to current medications, look for treatments and interventions based on new—but preliminary—understanding of mental illness, e.g., inflammation or other causes.

New is always exciting, but a silver bullet is unlikely. You'll approach anything new as another item to potentially add to your living treatment plan. It's another intervention among many, and you'll weigh its applicability against other options. If you try it, be sure to evaluate it against what's most important: your own goals and symptoms.

Patient-Generated Data

You do your own banking, scan your own groceries, and record your daily steps and sleep. Tracking your own mental health is not a big leap. Don't be surprised if clinics will require all their patients to fill out scales online between appointments, or use mood tracking apps or devices. They'll have more data to work with, which could be used to identify problems early on, leading to changes in your treatment plan.

If everyone is required to track their mental health, details specific to your own situation may be missed. Since you're already monitoring your own mental health, you know what measurements to focus on and how to interpret changes. You won't agree to treatment changes based on one simple measure if you know something else is a factor. You've practiced how to assertively but respectfully communicate with your treatment providers to ensure that point comes across.

Standardized Care

Clinic software already requires providers to collect more data at each appointment, even if it's not needed for clinical care. That takes a big chunk of time out of most peoples' appointments.

You, however, know the time and information challenges faced by mental health professionals and can help them simplify these tasks. You'll come prepared to your appointment with answers they can enter quickly. You'll work together to balance the time in your appointments, getting over the routine parts as quickly as possible. Still, with less time, it will be even more critical for you to prepare ahead and provide direction to get the most out of every appointment.

Reduced Care

The sustainability of the health care system is a growing concern. This will lead to even less time with specialists, and more of your care handled in routine ways by less expensive care providers. With the increasing demand for mental health care, this trend won't stop anytime soon.

This likely isn't a good thing, but you're well prepared to deal with it. Everything you've learned here has helped you help yourself in the face of limited or inadequate resources. You've got a huge head start.

More Options

Even if the basic level of mental health care available to the public is shrinking, there will always be extra services available for those who can afford them. Expect more privately paid, professional patient navigators specifically for mental health. It's already happening.[1] They'll offer a broader range of services addressing the entire spectrum of mental health care.

You already have the right attitude and skills. You wouldn't need to rely on such services for most of your care. Still, there may be small areas where you may want to access them. And, after all you now know and have gone through, you may find helping others to be an attractive career option.

Online Tools

With so much information shared online, look for new tools and technologies to help you maintain and share things such as your living treatment plan electronically.

Don't expect your care providers to start collaborating with you to maintain it. They're already overloaded, and privacy will remain a concern. Close sharing is still unnatural in health care. Likely, you'll share your plan with your care providers as you do now. Each has their unique area of emphasis, treatment style, and personality. You'll work with each one differently. What ties it together and makes it work is that you're in the centre. As you should be.

A Lifelong Journey

Improving your mental well-being is a lifelong journey. By practicing what you've learned here, and continuing to learn, you'll make the most of this journey. You'll increase your resilience in the face of further challenges. You're determined, and willing to be accountable for your own care. You listen, learn, respect others, and that attracts respect. You're persistent enough to get what you need, even if it's not always readily available. You are empowered. It's your mental health.

Connect With Us

Finally, we invite you to visit our website: mhnav.com.

There, you'll find a broad collection of tools and resources to complement this book, including updates and extras. It will also help you connect with us. Turn to *Appendix A* to learn more.

We'd love to hear about your own experiences with mental health care. What have you learned? What problems did you run into? Do you have any tips to share that could help others?

We look forward to hearing from you.

Appendices

A

Internet Resources

This appendix provides some reliable starting points when searching for additional information online.

Book Companion Website

First, please make sure to visit our website. It is a companion to this book. Consider this book as your starting point, and the website your next steps. You'll find bonus materials, additional resources, and opportunities to connect with us.

↪ https://mhnav.com/extras

Bonus Materials

On our website, you'll find additional original material we've written, beyond what's contained in this book.

For example, you'll see an in-depth article on the topic of mental health evidence, its limitations, how to apply and interpret it, common pitfalls, and more. It's an extension of the *Lies, Damn Lies, and Evidence* section found in the *Paging Dr. Google* chapter.

We'll also maintain a list of errata, corrections, and minor updates to the book. If you noticed any mistakes, please let us know.

Resources

Our website also includes an ever-expanding, up-to-date curated list of additional mental health tools and resources from around the web. The web sites listed shortly are only a starting point.

We want to make it easy for you to find the best, most relevant material. For example, you'll find recommended self-report scales for various mental illnesses. We also suggest selected workbooks that help you learn skills on your own to manage your symptoms.

Connect

Our website will also help you connect with us. We'd love to hear from you!

- Do you have comments or questions about what you've read?
- What did you learn when you applied this book to your situation?
- Is there anything you'd like to see either as bonus material on our website or in a future edition of this book?

Please sign up for our email list. You'll be the first to know about new tools and resources to help in your mental health journey.

You can also watch our blog. We'll post book and website updates and additions, mental health news, additional commentary, and more.

As a reminder, we can't provide medical advice specific to your situation. Please consult a physician for matters relating to your health and any symptoms that may require diagnosis or medical attention.

Other Sites

As noted, here are just a few sources that provide reliable mental health information. You'll find many more on our website, as described above.

Research

You learned about Google Scholar in the *Paging Dr. Google* chapter. Unlike a regular Google web search, it searches articles published in academic journals, conferences, and similar publications, including much of the PubMed database of biomedical literature. Full-text copies of many articles are available online, with citations and abstracts for the rest. It helps you get a sense of the context and importance of the article you're reading.

↪ https://scholar.google.com

If you're after a high-quality and reliable examination of the clinical evidence used to make important decisions, Cochrane is the place to start. Relevant research, methodologies and results are analyzed, providing you with a concise summary. Interventions are recommended only if high-quality evidence supports them. This can be subtly nuanced. Remember, too, the oft-quoted aphorism "the absence of evidence is not evidence of absence."

↪ https://cochrane.org

Medications

Your doctors and pharmacists should be your primary sources of information about medications, as they can take into account your unique health profile. For less personalized information, there are good sources available. In particular, both of these consumer-oriented sites contain detailed information on most medications (and many natural supplements). This includes approved and off-label uses, dosages, side effects, and warnings about potential serious consequences.

Both can identify potential medication (sometimes called "drug-drug") interactions. This can be useful when considering adding a new medication or supplement to your existing regimen. Potential interactions, no matter the severity, need to be interpreted by your doctor. They can take into account your overall health history, current symptoms, and previous treatment responses. Don't entirely rule out any medication based only on a potential interaction flagged by sites like these.

↪ https://drugs.com
↪ https://rxlist.com

Treatment Guidelines

There is an abundance of information that practitioners need to consider when creating a treatment plan. Psychiatrists David Goldbloom and Jon Davine compiled the essential information into a handbook aimed at helping family doctors provide the best evidence-based care for their patients with mental illness. *Psychiatry in Primary Care: A Concise Canadian Pocket Guide* is available in book and online form.

This guide includes practical information about each illness, including approaches to diagnosis, screening tools, treatment recommendations with links to full clinical guidelines, information on individual treatments, and many additional resources.

↪ https://www.porticonetwork.ca/web/psychiatry-primary-care

General Information

We can recommend several websites if you're looking for a broad range of reliable mental health information vetted by reputable organizations.

↪ https://mentalhealth.gov
↪ https://nimh.nih.gov
↪ https://camh.ca

Consumer Sites

These popular consumer sites aggregate a variety of mental health information, including news, articles, blogs, opinion pieces and more. Both have a large community of users. While neither is a good source for objective medical advice, many people who wish to engage in conversations about mental health find them helpful.
- ↪ https://healthyplace.com
- ↪ https://psychcentral.com

B

Talk Therapies

We provided a broad overview of psychotherapies in the *Talk Therapy* chapter. We showed you what therapy can look like. We described general categories of talk therapies and their goals, and how to use them as part of your living treatment plan.

This appendix provides an overview of several commonly-used, evidence-based talk therapies. Consider it a starting point used to discover which therapies might be helpful for you.

Most therapeutic modalities are applied to many different problems and illnesses, while some only work in specific situations. As with any treatment, your therapist should use them in a way that fits your overall treatment goals. You should also regularly measure your progress toward those goals during a course of therapy.

There are many more talk therapies than we cover here. The Psychology Today and GoodTherapy websites describe many types of therapies:
  ↪ https://www.psychologytoday.com/types-of-therapy
  ↪ https://www.goodtherapy.org/learn-about-therapy/types

Cognitive Behavioural Therapy (CBT)

CBT is a short-term, goal-oriented collection of psychotherapeutic techniques. It is based on the premise that your thoughts, feelings, and behaviours all affect each other. Changing unhealthy patterns in the way you think (thoughts) or behave can positively influence your mood (feelings).

Learning and practicing CBT techniques help you "rewire" your brain, building new connections between neurons. Imaging studies have observed brain changes as a result of CBT. Practicing is key, so active participation both during and between sessions (i.e., homework) is crucial. It is a very well-studied therapy that can be as effective as medication in some situations. Often, a combination of CBT and medication is optimal.

There are dozens of different CBT techniques. You need to choose the right techniques to use and the right thoughts or behaviours to work on. Two people suffering from depression, who undergo CBT, may work on completely different things using completely different techniques. CBT techniques have been successfully applied to a vast range of symptoms, e.g., depression, panic, compulsions, insomnia, binge eating, pain. We'll now briefly examine three categories of CBT techniques.

Cognitive Restructuring

Changing the way you think is called cognitive restructuring. Like most people, you likely have thoughts that automatically pop into your mind at different times. Some may be distorted and not based on reality, e.g., "I am worthless." These can negatively affect your mood and behaviour. CBT techniques help you identify these thoughts, challenge them, and replace them with balanced alternatives based on reality. With practice, these changes become ingrained. Gradually, these changes in your thoughts improve your mood and change your behaviour. Breaking down this process:

- *Thought records* and *mood logs* capture automatic thoughts for analysis.
- Automatic thoughts are examined for a wide range of logical errors called *cognitive distortions,* e.g., all-or-none thinking, overgeneralization, jumping to conclusions.
- Evidence both for and against automatic thoughts is collected and reviewed.
- Based on refuting cognitive distortions, assessing evidence, or other techniques like pros-and-cons, more balanced thoughts are generated.

Exposure

As cognitive restructuring helps to change automatic thoughts, exposure helps to change automatic behaviours like avoidance. People avoid things that may contribute to their anxiety. The anxious mind overestimates the negative consequences of being around people or objects, in situations, or doing activities. Exposure makes you repeatedly face the things you've been avoiding. Your confidence increases each time you successfully expose yourself to a trigger. This decreases your avoidance and positively affects your thoughts, mood and anxiety.

For exposure activities to be successful, you start with less anxiety-provoking situations, and gradually introduce situations associated with increasing anxiety. For example, addressing a phobia of snakes might involve reading about snakes, then looking at pictures of snakes, holding a toy snake, looking at a small snake at a pet store, and several more steps before eventually holding a snake. Exposure can be done via:

- facing the object, situation or activity in real life, known as *in vivo* exposure;
- imagining an object, situation or activity, known as *imaginal* exposure;
- bringing on physical sensations associated with the anxiety (e.g., shortness of breath) when the object, situation or activity is not present, known as *interoceptive* exposure; and
- using other techniques, e.g., virtual reality.

Behavioural Activation (BA)

When you are emotionally overwhelmed, you're less likely to take part in activities that you enjoy. You tend to isolate and detach from others. You avoid things that will likely improve your mood. You'd rather stay in bed. Your symptoms worsen, leading to more avoidance—a vicious circle.

Behavioural activation forces you to do things that you enjoy, to eventually improve your feelings and thoughts. Some notable aspects:

- Activities are rigidly scheduled, usually on a weekly basis, and defined very precisely; you can easily say if you've completed an activity or not.
- Detailed planning helps avoid relying on motivation; in fact, you're using behaviour to improve motivation and not vice versa.
- Activities are chosen that are consistent with your values and are important to you (not others), bringing pleasure or a sense of accomplishment.
- Mood charting helps identify activities that you enjoy and to monitor your mood between activities.
- As with exposure, you start with smaller and less intimidating activities, gradually progressing to activities that you are more strongly compelled to avoid.

Other Skills and Techniques

Several other therapeutic skills and techniques are commonly used, either standalone or incorporated into CBT or other therapies.

Mindfulness

Mindfulness is a broad set of practices that help you remain in the here-and-now and decrease your baseline stress level. Adapted from Buddhist meditation practices, many modern forms of mindfulness have good clinical evidence supporting them. Typical mindfulness exercises include forms of meditation, visualization, body scans, and being in the present when performing activities like eating. These exercises teach and enhance five core skills:

- *Observe.* Notice things that are happening both inside and outside you.
- *Describe.* Organize and convey what you are aware of at the moment.
- *Detach.* Allow thoughts, feelings, memories and sensations to simply be present without becoming absorbed in mental evaluation—"letting go."
- *Self-compassion.* Practice acceptance, care and kindness to yourself. Accept yourself, flaws and all.
- *Act mindfully.* Act with intention, reflecting your beliefs and principles in the present moment.

Mindfulness is a general skill applied to many illnesses and often combined with other therapies. Notable variations include mindfulness-based cognitive therapy (MBCT) and mindfulness-based stress reduction (MBSR).

Psychoeducation and Bibliotherapy

These are the fancy terms for reading and using self-help materials. Psychoeducation helps you understand your illness and learn techniques to improve your symptoms. Reading this book is a good example. You can find many good books on almost any mental health topic. Workbooks (and to some degree, apps for various devices) also provide exercises to help practice different techniques. Though primarily a solo form of therapy, treatment providers can play valuable roles, recommending resources, encouraging you, and monitoring your progress to help you stay engaged, accountable, and on track.

Relaxation

A wide range of practices can help you relax and decrease stress. They are often incorporated into psychotherapy programs. These help a variety of physical and mental health problems. Many of the mindfulness techniques promote relaxation. Other examples include deep breathing, biofeedback, meditation, yoga, massage, acupuncture, reflexology, T'ai chi, Qigong, flotation therapy, and taking a walk in the park. Admittedly, we may be stretching the boundaries of *talk* therapy pretty far with some of these.

Other Therapies

Here, we note some of the other more commonly used therapies. Remember that these are only a small fraction of those available, and each therapy has many variations.

Problem-Solving Therapy (PST)

Problem-solving therapy uses a cognitive-behavioural approach to help you learn and improve problem-solving skills. It also helps increase your optimism and acceptance to enhance your problem-solving and healthy coping. This therapy has been widely applied to a variety of stressors and psychological problems.

In PST, you define problems, come up with potential solutions, decide amongst the alternatives, and then implement and evaluate the chosen solution. You explore practical barriers to problem-solving (e.g., ambiguity or conflicting goals), negative problem-solving styles (e.g., avoidance or impulsivity) and other mental obstacles (e.g., cognitive overload, poor motivation, decreased emotional regulation).

Interpersonal Psychotherapy (IPT)

Interpersonal psychotherapy helps you understand the connection between the onset and fluctuation of your symptoms and a recent challenge in your life, e.g., relationships. You use that information to find ways of dealing with the life challenge, thereby improving your symptoms. Therapists offer support and ideas for change. IPT is usually highly structured, with a course of therapy usually lasting 12-16 weeks. IPT can help with:

- grief and loss;
- interpersonal role disputes, typically conflict with another person leading to tension and distress;

- life changes and role transitions, such as losing a job, the birth of a child, starting a new relationship; and
- challenges with interpersonal skills that make it difficult to start or sustain relationships.

IPT is most often used for forms of depression and bipolar disorders. Interpersonal and social rhythm therapy (IPSRT) is a notable variation.

Acceptance and Commitment Therapy (ACT)

ACT is a short-term, practical, down-to-earth form of therapy. It combines mindfulness with tools to modify behaviour.

When faced with negative experiences that you can't change (e.g., illness, end of a relationship), ACT encourages you to accept reality without analyzing or trying to control the situation. Struggling often leads to overreaction, obsession, and avoidance. ACT teaches you how to observe your current reaction and gain control over it. Through a series of skills and strategies, you learn to identify and then choose alternative ways of reacting that are consistent with your values. You set goals and commit to your chosen set of actions. So:

- Accept your reactions and be present.
- Choose a valued direction.
- Take action.

Like CBT, ACT has been widely used to treat many different illnesses.

Dialectical Behaviour Therapy (DBT)

DBT is a multifaceted program used to help those who frequently experience intense emotion, which can lead to impulsive behaviour, self-harm, and substance use. It was initially designed to treat borderline personality disorder but has been used, in whole or in part, for depression, PTSD, binge eating and addiction.

A full DBT program is typically one year long, mixing individual and group psychotherapy and skills training. Many smaller programs focus on specific subsets and skills. Several individual skills and techniques developed within DBT, e.g., grounding techniques, have also been incorporated into other therapies.

Like ACT, DBT begins with accepting emotions and situations. It then proceeds through the process of change. Tools, techniques and coping skills are divided into four modules:

- mindfulness (observe and describe emotions, withholding judgment, focus);
- interpersonal effectiveness (assertiveness, communication);
- distress tolerance (grounding, relaxation, self-soothing, distraction); and
- emotional regulation (understanding emotion, problem-solving, health).

Psychodynamic Therapies

Psychodynamic therapy is a form of insight-oriented psychotherapy. Here, you explore your past to gain a better understanding of your current behaviours in order to change them. Its focus on the past separates it from most modern therapies that are entirely forward-looking. It is a modern evolution of Freudian psychoanalysis.

Full psychodynamic therapy is extremely open-ended, wide-ranging, and lengthy. Short-term variations are briefer (weeks or months versus years), more focused, and thereby more practical for most people. While few therapists practice pure psychodynamic therapy, many incorporate some aspects and interpretations into more eclectic mixtures of therapies when treating various symptoms. Psychodynamic concepts are also used by therapists when formulating a patient's presentation.

Supportive Psychotherapy

Supportive psychotherapy aims to improve symptoms via a therapist's positive, respectful and optimistic engagement with you. This general approach increases your comfort in sharing personal information and reduces your anxiety. It can help boost your self-esteem while developing new skills to address symptoms. Therapists commonly:

- demonstrate support, acceptance, and warmth toward you;
- emphasize how they will work collaboratively with you;
- are optimistic and hopeful that your goals will be met;
- help you normalize, clarify or reframe experiences in a more positive light;
- respect your defences and boundaries;
- offer advice and teach you new skills; and
- focus on your strengths and give positive feedback on growth.

Humanistic

Humanistic therapies help you to identify and fulfill your unique purpose and potential as a whole individual. They take a holistic approach rooted in personal self-awareness and experience in the present moment, not the past. The therapist's role is to create a positive and empathetic environment for you to share feelings; they do not act as an authority figure.

Common variations of these therapies include client-centred therapy, existential psychotherapy, and Gestalt therapy.

Eye Movement Desensitization and Reprocessing (EMDR)

EMDR was designed to treat posttraumatic stress and has been applied to help deal with other distressing life events. Some memories can remain *unprocessed* due to the distress present at the time of the event. They stay stored in your brain as raw emotion and are not incorporated into the complex structure of your personal story. Future events that are in some way associated with the unprocessed memory cause you to respond as you did to the original event.

An EMDR therapist helps you reprocess those original distressing unresolved memories. They ask you to remember the unprocessed memory and focus on an external stimulus that the therapist provides. Your eyes move side-to-side, following the horizontal movement of the therapist's finger (hence the name of the therapy). The therapist then asks you to shift your thoughts to more positive ideas or images. This helps weaken the strong negative associations of the original memory.

While there's little understanding of how bilateral stimulus helps (other stimuli are also used), the therapy can effectively help you deal with past trauma.

C

Medications

The medication chapters in this book provided general information about several classes of psychotropic medications.

With that knowledge in mind, this appendix provides an introduction to specific medications within these general classes. For each medication, we list basic information and share what we consider are the things that differentiate it from other medications in the same class. This will help you begin to compare your options. Some of the resources mentioned in Appendix A will give much greater detail.

Here are a few things to keep in mind in order to make the best use of this material.

Medication selection. We only include a subset of the several dozen psychotropic medications in use today. We've chosen those that are either commonly used or are particularly effective for specific problems. Most of these are off-patent. Relatively affordable generic versions are available as well as brand-name ones. They've also been on the market long enough that their benefits and risks have been monitored over time.

Uses. Each medication is most commonly used for a particular set of illnesses based on formal and informal clinical experiences. There are two important caveats. First, just because an illness is on the list doesn't mean that the medication will help you with that illness. Second, even if an illness is not on the list, the medication may help you with that illness.

Approvals. You've likely heard the terms *approved for* or *indicated for* applied to medications. These mean that a pharmaceutical company has supplied acceptable evidence to a government regulator (e.g., the FDA or Health Canada) showing that the medication can help with the given problem. Often this evidence comes from clinical trials carried out by the pharmaceutical company. These usually involve at least several hundred patients and take place before the medication is approved in a country.

Not every use for a medication is officially government-approved. Many medications have shown to be very useful for conditions other than those approved by government regulators. Such use is termed *off-label*. Using a medication off-label is not wrong. Yes, there may be little evidence suggesting it will work. But, there could be strong evidence saying it is helpful, but nobody went through the time-consuming and expensive process of getting government approval. Ask why it's being recommended in your case.

Approvals also vary by country—we'll note official approvals in Canada and the USA. Sometimes only one version of a medication is approved even though it comes in multiple forms (usually the newest one the pharmaceutical company is actively marketing). We'll note this with a '†'.

Actions. We note the main neurotransmitters that each medication affects. This only begins to tell the story. Medications act on those neurotransmitters and their receptors in many different ways. Most also have additional effects on other neurotransmitters not mentioned.

Sources. Product monographs are detailed documents prepared by pharmaceutical companies. They are required by regulators (e.g., Health Canada, FDA) and can be considered the official story.

When it comes to combining evidence-based data and real-world use, we have generally deferred to *Stahl's Essential Psychopharmacology: Prescriber's Guide (sixth edition)* by Dr. Stephen Stahl.

Antidepressants

The first category of medications is antidepressants. As you'll recall, these help with not only depression and anxiety but a range of other concerns including impulsivity, skin picking, chronic pain, premature ejaculation, and gastrointestinal distress due to irritable bowel syndrome.

Fluoxetine (Prozac)

TYPE	USED FOR
selective serotonin reuptake inhibitor (SSRI)	major depressive disorder[US,CA]
	obsessive-compulsive disorder[US,CA]
	premenstrual dysphoric disorder[US]
ACTS ON	bulimia nervosa[US,CA]
serotonin	panic disorder[US]
	social anxiety disorder
	posttraumatic stress disorder

Fluoxetine was the first of the "new generation" of antidepressants to reach the mainstream market (in 1987) and is still in common use today.

Fluoxetine has the longest half-life of current generation antidepressants. After stopping it, it takes up to seven weeks to leave your system, whereas most take two weeks. This leads to minimal withdrawal if any. It's suitable for people who sometimes miss medication doses. It's also often prescribed to reduce withdrawal symptoms when tapering off other antidepressants.

It's most commonly available in capsule and liquid form. Most people find it stimulating, and therefore take it in the morning.

Paroxetine (Paxil)

TYPE	USED FOR
selective serotonin reuptake inhibitor (SSRI)	major depressive disorder[US,CA]
	obsessive-compulsive disorder[USt,CA]
	panic disorder[USt,CA]
ACTS ON	social anxiety disorder[US,CA]
serotonin	generalized anxiety disorder[USt,CA]
	posttraumatic stress disorder[USt,CA]
	premenstrual dysphoric disorder[USt]

Paroxetine is often used to treat depression in those who also have anxiety. Side effects like weight gain and sedation can be experienced more frequently than with other SSRIs. Paroxetine is associated with significant withdrawal symptoms. Questions regarding its safety in pregnancy (possible increased risk of cardiovascular malformation) are being explored.

Citalopram (Celexa)

TYPE	USED FOR
selective serotonin reuptake inhibitor (SSRI)	depression[US,CA]
	obsessive-compulsive disorder
	panic disorder
ACTS ON	social anxiety disorder
serotonin	generalized anxiety disorder
	posttraumatic stress disorder
	premenstrual dysphoric disorder

Citalopram is generally well tolerated and has relatively few medication interactions. Because of this, it is well-studied and frequently used in people with physical illness taking several other medications. Doses above 40mg carry an increased risk of lengthening the heart's QTc interval. Escitalopram is very similar to citalopram.

Escitalopram (Cipralex, Lexapro)

TYPE
selective serotonin reuptake inhibitor (SSRI)

ACTS ON
serotonin

USED FOR
major depressive disorder[US,CA]
generalized anxiety disorder[US,CA]
obsessive-compulsive disorder[CA]
panic disorder
social anxiety disorder
posttraumatic stress disorder
premenstrual dysphoric disorder

Escitalopram is a newer (went generic in 2012) and cleaner version of citalopram, which was itself already a well-tolerated medication with few interactions. Escitalopram improves on both of these aspects, with an even lower incidence of most side effects and even fewer medication interactions. A dose of escitalopram is equivalent to twice that dose of citalopram. Monitoring the heart's QTc interval is needed above 20mg, though the medication can be used up to 40mg in most cases.

Despite their similarities, some people find that either citalopram or escitalopram is effective and well-tolerated, but not the other.

Sertraline (Zoloft)

TYPE
selective serotonin reuptake inhibitor (SSRI)

ACTS ON
serotonin

USED FOR
major depressive disorder[US,CA]
obsessive-compulsive disorder[US,CA]
panic disorder[US,CA]
social anxiety disorder[US]
premenstrual dysphoric disorder[US]
posttraumatic stress disorder[US]
generalized anxiety disorder

Sertraline is another well-studied, well-tolerated medication with few interactions. Notably, it was found to be safe in studies of patients with cardiovascular disease. Sertraline is absorbed 25% better when taken with food.

Fluvoxamine (Luvox)

TYPE
selective serotonin reuptake inhibitor (SSRI)

ACTS ON
serotonin

USED FOR
obsessive-compulsive disorder[US,CA]
depression[CA]
social anxiety disorder[US†]
panic disorder
posttraumatic stress disorder
generalized anxiety disorder

Fluvoxamine is used for depression and anxiety. It is especially effective in treating obsessive-compulsive disorder (OCD), second only to clomipramine.

It has a low incidence of sexual side effects, though it can cause nausea. It has more potential medication interactions than many other SSRIs. Smoking slows its removal through the liver by 25%, thereby increasing its blood level.

Venlafaxine (Effexor)

TYPE	USED FOR
serotonin norepinephrine reuptake inhibitor (SNRI)	major depressive disorder[US,CA]
	generalized anxiety disorder[US,CA]
	social anxiety disorder[US,CA]
ACTS ON	panic disorder[US,CA]
serotonin, norepinephrine, dopamine (weakly)	posttraumatic stress disorder
	premenstrual dysphoric disorder

For most people, venlafaxine primarily affects serotonin at lower doses. From 150mg upwards, it affects both serotonin and norepinephrine, and from 225mg upwards, there is a small dopamine contribution.

Above 150mg, it targets symptoms like concentration, motivation, and energy that do not respond as well to SSRIs. It can have a severe discontinuation syndrome, emphasizing the need to stop it very slowly and gradually, in collaboration with your doctor.

While an immediate-release version was first introduced, today, the once-daily extended-release form is used almost exclusively. Venlafaxine can cause hypertension.

Desvenlafaxine (Pristiq)

TYPE	USED FOR
serotonin-norepinephrine reuptake inhibitor (SNRI)	major depressive disorder[US,CA]
	generalized anxiety disorder
	social anxiety disorder
ACTS ON	panic disorder
serotonin, norepinephrine, dopamine (weakly)	posttraumatic stress disorder
	premenstrual dysphoric disorder
	fibromyalgia

Desvenlafaxine is the "next generation" of venlafaxine. Venlafaxine is metabolized into desvenlafaxine by the liver. This newer medication skips this step, so it is not influenced by the CYP450 system or liver disease.

Dosing options (50mg or 100mg tablets) are limited, and the tablets cannot be split without affecting the continuous release mechanism. The 50mg dose affects both serotonin and norepinephrine. Doses above 100mg generally provide little added symptom relief, though side effects increase.

As with venlafaxine, withdrawal symptoms can be severe. If you have problems reducing below the lowest dose of 50mg, you can switch to venlafaxine (desvenlafaxine 50mg ≈ venlafaxine 150mg), which can be reduced more gradually. Alternatively, short-acting low dose desvenlafaxine can be compounded and taken twice daily. Fluoxetine can also be added to decrease withdrawal symptoms.

Duloxetine (Cymbalta)

TYPE
serotonin-norepinephrine reuptake inhibitor (SNRI)

ACTS ON
serotonin, norepinephrine, dopamine (weakly)

USED FOR
major depressive disorder[US,CA]
generalized anxiety disorder[US,CA]
fibromyalgia[US,CA]
diabetic peripheral neuropathic pain[US,CA]
chronic musculoskeletal pain[US,CA]
other anxiety disorders
stress urinary incontinence

Duloxetine generally has a lower incidence of problematic side effects and withdrawal symptoms than venlafaxine (the other main SNRI).

Duloxetine works on both serotonin and norepinephrine at the 30mg dose. Doses above 60mg show a greater incremental effect on norepinephrine and dopamine. Dose options are limited in Canada (30mg, 60mg), though a 20mg option is also available in the USA.

For more flexibility, doses of any size can be halved by opening up the capsule and splitting the enteric-coated pellets between the halves. Each half is then sealed, e.g., with a bit of bread or soft cheese. Alternatively, half of the pellets can be added to applesauce, which has the correct pH to maintain the extended-release properties.

Mirtazapine (Remeron)

TYPE
noradrenaline and specific serotonin agent (NaSSA)

ACTS ON
serotonin, norepinephrine

USED FOR
major depressive disorder[US,CA]
generalized anxiety disorder
panic disorder
posttraumatic stress disorder

The medications we've described so far work by inhibiting neurotransmitter reuptake. In contrast, mirtazapine uses a novel mechanism to influence various neurotransmitter receptors. This leads to an increase in serotonin and norepinephrine.

It often helps insomnia and anxiety more quickly than other antidepressants, and its effect can be slightly faster than SSRIs on depressive symptoms. Unlike the SSRIs and SNRIs, it generally does not cause sexual side effects.

Increased appetite leading to weight gain is frequent. Mirtazapine helps those experiencing brain induced nausea due to anxiety or physical illness. It uses the same mechanism as ondansetron, an anti-nausea medication commonly given alongside chemotherapy. Flu-like symptoms (indicating a decreased white blood count), hypotension, and sedation can also occur.

Bupropion (Wellbutrin)

TYPE
noradrenaline and dopamine reuptake inhibitor (NDRI)

ACTS ON
norepinephrine, dopamine

USED FOR
major depressive disorder[US,CA]
nicotine addiction[US,CA]
seasonal affective disorder[US†,CA†]
bipolar depression
attention-deficit hyperactivity disorder
sexual dysfunction

Bupropion is the first medication we're describing that works on norepinephrine and dopamine, but *not serotonin*. Most people use the once-daily extended-release version, as opposed to the immediate (three times a day) or sustained (twice a day) version. The latter is used most commonly to change dosages.

Bupropion is frequently added to an SSRI to help with antidepressant-induced sexual dysfunction, as well as provide other benefits. It treats cognitive symptoms of depression, as well as apathy. Bupropion has a lower likelihood than SSRIs of inducing hypomania or mania if a bipolar disorder is suspected.

It will often *increase anxiety and irritability,* more commonly than the other antidepressants we've described so far. Bupropion has a small risk of inducing a seizure (0.4% versus ≤0.1% for SSRIs/SNRIs) and this risk increases to 4% at doses over 450mg. It should not be used if alcohol abuse or withdrawal is an issue, if you've had an eating disorder, or if you're already at risk for seizure.

Bupropion is the same medication marketed as Zyban for smoking cessation.

Amitriptyline (Elavil)

TYPE
tricyclic antidepressant (TCA)

ACTS ON
serotonin, norepinephrine

USED FOR
depression[US,CA]
neuropathic or chronic pain
back or neck pain
fibromyalgia
headache
anxiety
insomnia

Amitriptyline is one of the most popular *tricyclics*, which are the generation of antidepressants that immediately preceded today's SSRIs and others. It is still widely used, both for severe or treatment-resistant depression and for a variety of chronic physical conditions. Amitriptyline is metabolized into nortriptyline.

When taking a tricyclic, tell your doctor about all of your health conditions, prescribed medications, and supplements. Severe interactions with other medications and natural supplements can occur. Tricyclics can worsen some cardiac and other physical health conditions. They are not safe in pregnancy.

Nortriptyline (Aventyl, Pamelor)

TYPE
tricyclic antidepressant (TCA)

ACTS ON
serotonin, norepinephrine

USED FOR
depression[US,CA]
neuropathic or chronic pain
anxiety
insomnia

Another tricyclic, your body converts amitriptyline into nortriptyline. The two medications are very similar, both used for treatment-resistant depression and chronic pain. Nortriptyline can be combined with an SSRI to improve cognitive symptoms and apathy. Medication levels can be monitored through simple blood tests, which can help optimize your dosage. It is usually better tolerated than amitriptyline.

See the previous note on amitriptyline regarding tricyclics, medication interactions, and safety.

Clomipramine (Anafranil)

TYPE
tricyclic antidepressant (TCA)

ACTS ON
serotonin, norepinephrine

USED FOR
obsessive-compulsive disorder[US,CA]
depression[CA]
neuropathic or chronic pain
anxiety
insomnia

Clomipramine is a tricyclic antidepressant used for OCD, and to a lesser degree, severe depression. Clomipramine is considered the "gold standard" (most effective) treatment for OCD. However, SSRIs are often tried first because they generally have fewer side effects. Like nortriptyline, its level can be monitored with blood tests to help optimize the dose.

See the previous note on amitriptyline regarding tricyclics, medication interactions, and safety.

Other Antidepressants

We have included three of the older tricyclic antidepressants that are in common use. There are several others available that are often used in specific situations.

Another broad category of antidepressants is monoamine oxidase inhibitors (MAOIs), whose period of peak use overlapped tricyclics. MAOIs like phenelzine (Nardil) and tranylcypromine (Parnate) are used today, usually when other medications have failed. Most (but not all) require being on a low tyramine diet to prevent a hypertensive crisis. This makes them less appealing to most people.

A few newer antidepressants have been released in recent years. Vilazodone (Viibryd) works on serotonin using a different mechanism than existing medications. Vortioxetine (Trintellix) takes a different approach by targeting multiple neurotransmitters, though can cause severe nausea. Finally, levomilnacipran (Fetzima) is a new SNRI, the same class as venlafaxine or duloxetine. All of these new medications are approved for treating depression. They are used for other illnesses as well.

Other classes of medications are often used to augment antidepressants, helping to address particular symptoms, or boosting the effectiveness of the antidepressant. These include mood stabilizers, sedatives and hypnotics, antipsychotics and stimulants—in other words, everything else!

Sedatives and Hypnotics

The next category of psychotropic medications is sedatives (which help reduce anxiety) and hypnotics (which help with sleep). Most of these medications (e.g., benzodiazepines) can help on a short-term or "as needed" basis. As you'll recall from the *Other Medications* chapter, they are not used long term as they can affect memory, balance, and reaction time. They are associated with tolerance and withdrawal. For longer-term control of anxiety, other medications (e.g., antidepressants or antipsychotics) are preferred.

Alprazolam (Xanax)

TYPE
benzodiazepine (anxiolytic)

ACTS ON
GABA

USED FOR
generalized anxiety disorder[US†,CA]
panic disorder[US]
other anxiety disorders
anxiety associated with depression
premenstrual dysphoric disorder
somatic symptoms of anxiety disorders
insomnia
catatonia

Alprazolam is one of the most commonly used anxiolytics, particularly in the USA. It works within 15-30mins, but the effect only lasts a few hours. This makes it a good "as needed" medication. For continuous anxiety, it should be taken at least three times a day, sometimes more, to prevent withdrawal between doses. Withdrawal can cause increased anxiety, called rebound anxiety. A longer-acting, extended-release (XR) version of alprazolam is also available in the USA.

Lorazepam (Ativan)

TYPE
benzodiazepine (anxiolytic, anticonvulsant)

ACTS ON
GABA

USED FOR
anxiety disorder[US,CA]
anxiety associated with depression[US]
insomnia
muscle spasm
alcohol withdrawal psychosis
headache
panic disorder
catatonia

Lorazepam is another short-acting benzodiazepine, which has a fairly wide variety of uses beyond its main use of treating acute anxiety. It's more commonly used for episodic anxiety in Canada than in the USA, where alprazolam is more popular. Oral, sublingual, intramuscular and intravenous forms are available. It also takes effect quickly, and only lasts several hours, making it a good "as needed" medication. It, too, requires multiple daily doses for ongoing anxiety.

Clonazepam (Klonopin, Rivotril)

TYPE
benzodiazepine (anxiolytic, anticonvulsant)

ACTS ON
GABA

USED FOR
panic disorder[US]
akinetic, myoclonic, absence seizures[US,CA]
other seizures
other anxiety disorders
insomnia
catatonia

Clonazepam lasts approximately six hours. This is considerably longer than either alprazolam or lorazepam. This makes it a good fit for ongoing anxiety, where using shorter-acting medications may lead to withdrawal and increased anxiety before the next dose. It is also used to help you fall and stay asleep.

Diazepam (Valium)

TYPE
benzodiazepine (anxiolytic, muscle relaxant, anticonvulsant)

ACTS ON
GABA

USED FOR
anxiety disorder[US,CA]
symptoms of anxiety (short-term)[US,CA]
acute alcohol withdrawal[US,CA]
certain muscle spasms[US,CA]
insomnia
catatonia

Diazepam stays working in your system for several days, and so is very forgiving around the timing of dosages. It, too, is useful for extended periods of anxiety. If you are having difficulty withdrawing from other benzodiazepines, the preferred approach is to switch to diazepam and slowly reduce its dose (see Dr. Ashton's benzo website, benzo.org.uk). Diazepam is available in pill and intravenous forms.

Zolpidem (Ambien, Sublinox)

TYPE
non-benzodiazepine hypnotic

ACTS ON
GABA

USED FOR
short-term treatment of insomnia[US,CA]

Zolpidem and other "z-drugs" work similarly to benzodiazepines but are considered somewhat safer. They are still intended for short term use. Short- and long-acting versions of zolpidem are available. Some people report periods of amnesia between when they take the medication and when they fall asleep. Sleepwalking and other behaviours have occurred.

Zopiclone (Imovane)

TYPE
non-benzodiazepine hypnotic

USED FOR
short-term treatment of insomnia[CA]

ACTS ON
GABA

Zopiclone has very similar properties to zolpidem, described previously. Zopiclone is not commercially available in the United States, though the very similar eszopiclone is.

Eszopiclone (Lunesta)

TYPE
non-benzodiazepine hypnotic

ACTS ON
GABA

USED FOR
insomnia[US]
primary insomnia
chronic insomnia
transient insomnia
insomnia secondary to other conditions
insomnia following antidepressant treatment

Eszopiclone has very similar properties to zolpidem and zopiclone. Eszopiclone is such a close relative of zopiclone that some jurisdictions denied it patent protection as a unique medication. It is available in the United States. Though short-term use is recommended, technically, the FDA has approved it for longer-term use.

Trazodone (Desyrel)

TYPE
serotonin antagonist/reuptake inhibitor

ACTS ON
serotonin

USED FOR
depression[US,CA]
insomnia
anxiety

Technically an antidepressant, trazodone is rarely used for depression, as most people cannot tolerate its side effects at the high dose needed to improve depressive symptoms. It's most commonly used to help fall and stay asleep, though it should be avoided if a bipolar disorder is suspected. Assuming a sufficient dose, it will help with insomnia right away. It's an excellent alternative to more addictive hypnotics, as there is no development of tolerance, dependence, and limited withdrawal. It can be used over the long term. Postural hypotension can occur. Priapism (prolonged penile/clitoral erection) is a very rare side effect.

Buspirone (Buspar)

TYPE
serotonin receptor partial agonist; anxiolytic

ACTS ON
serotonin

USED FOR
management of anxiety disorders[US]
short-term treatment of symptoms of anxiety[US,CA]
mixed anxiety and depression

Buspirone is often combined with other medications to help with anxiety over the long term. While not a first-line agent, it has a favourable side-effect profile compared with most antidepressants and benzodiazepines. It does take a few weeks to have an effect. It is used either regularly or as-needed to mitigate the sexual side effects of antidepressants.

Pregabalin (Lyrica)

TYPE
gabapentinoid

ACTS ON
voltage-sensitive calcium channels

USED FOR
diabetic peripheral neuropathy[US,CA]
postherpetic neuralgia[US,CA]
fibromyalgia[US,CA]
neuropathic pain[US,CA]
generalized anxiety disorder
panic disorder
social anxiety disorder

Pregabalin, and its predecessor, gabapentin, are structurally similar to the neurotransmitter GABA and can cross the blood-brain barrier. Despite that, they don't actually affect GABA transmission but rely on a different mechanism altogether. Pregabalin can help with pain, as well as both psychological and physical symptoms of anxiety. It has approval in Europe for treating generalized anxiety disorder. Its effects are often felt in one week, faster than antidepressants, and it can be used long term. However, concerns about its abuse potential are beginning to surface. It has a favourable side-effect profile and a wide range of effective doses.

Propranolol (Inderal)

TYPE
beta-blocker, antihypertensive

ACTS ON
epinephrine, norepinephrine

USED FOR
migraine prophylaxis[US,CA]
essential tremor[US]
hypertension[US,CA]
various cardiac issues[US,CA]
violence, aggression
posttraumatic stress disorder
generalized anxiety disorder

While propranolol is primarily used to reduce blood pressure, it has a few very particular mental health benefits. It can help reduce symptoms of aggression and agitation and is used to decrease performance anxiety. It can reduce feelings of anger and being on edge associated with prior traumatic events, such as those associated with PTSD. It should be used carefully, as it can theoretically worsen depression and cause many physical effects.

Prazosin (Minipress)

TYPE
alpha-blocker, antihypertensive

ACTS ON
norepinephrine

USED FOR
hypertension[US,CA]
nightmares associated with PTSD

Prazosin is another blood pressure medication. It can help reduce nightmares, particularly those associated with posttraumatic stress disorder.

Mood Stabilizers

Mood stabilizers are generally a core component of the medication regime used to treat bipolar disorders.

Lithium

TYPE
mood stabilizer

ACTS ON
unknown and complex

USED FOR
manic episodes in bipolar disorder[US,CA]
maintenance therapy in bipolar 1 disorder [US,CA]
bipolar depression
major depressive disorder (augmenting agent)

One of the oldest and (chemically) simplest agents, lithium treats acute episodes of mania and depression and helps prevent further high or low mood states. It also significantly reduces suicidal thoughts. It is often paired with one of the anticonvulsant mood stabilizers, an antipsychotic, or (with caution) an antidepressant.

While effective, you need lab tests before starting and periodic lab tests while taking it. Avoiding dehydration and watching for signs of lithium toxicity are also necessary. The correct dosage is determined by blood levels, which can also be affected by other medications. Weight gain and sedation are also common. It is excreted by the kidney and does not depend on the liver at all. It is associated with mild–severe fetal cardiac abnormalities in pregnancy.

Valproic Acid (Depakote, Epival)

TYPE	**USED FOR**
mood stabilizer, anticonvulsant	manic episodes in bipolar disorder[US,CA]
	various types of seizures[US,CA]
ACTS ON	migraine prophylaxis[US†]
GABA, sodium channels, calcium channels	maintenance therapy in bipolar disorder
	bipolar depression

Many different formulations of this anticonvulsant are available. It is commonly used in those with bipolar disorders, assisting to keep manic symptoms in check. It can help with aggression, agitation, and impulsivity in other situations. You will need lab tests before starting it, more tests to find the right dosage, and then periodic tests to watch for early signs of long-term physical effects. Weight gain and sedation are common. It can cause fetal neural tube defects in pregnancy, though a folic acid supplement can reduce this risk.

Carbamazepine (Tegretol)

TYPE	**USED FOR**
mood stabilizer, anticonvulsant	manic episodes in bipolar disorder[US,CA]
	various types of seizures[US,CA]
ACTS ON	maintenance therapy in bipolar disorder
GABA, sodium channels, glutamate	bipolar depression

Carbamazepine was the first anticonvulsant widely used to treat bipolar disorders. It also requires lab tests before starting, more tests to find the right dosage, and periodic monitoring for physical effects thereafter. Weight gain is slightly less problematic than with lithium or valproic acid. It is very sedating. It decreases the effectiveness of hormonal contraception. It can cause fetal neural tube defects in pregnancy, though a folic acid supplement can reduce this risk. There is a rare chance of experiencing a severe rash (see lamotrigine, next).

Extended-release versions (e.g., Tegretol CR) and a successor medication, oxcarbazepine (Trileptal) are overall better tolerated by many people.

Lamotrigine (Lamictal)

TYPE	**USED FOR**
mood stabilizer, anticonvulsant	various types of seizures[US,CA]
	maintenance therapy in bipolar disorder[US]
ACTS ON	bipolar depression
sodium channels, calcium channels, glutamate, aspartate	bipolar mania
	neuropathic and chronic pain
	major depressive disorder

Compared to lithium, valproic acid, and carbamazepine, lamotrigine is very well tolerated. It has a lower incidence of side effects and little tendency toward weight gain or sedation. Lab tests are not required either before or during use, though its blood level is decreased with hormonal contraception. It is more effective in treating acute depressive symptoms, so is used for bipolar depression and less commonly for unipolar depression with anxiety.

There is a rare possibility (<0.1%) of developing a rash that, if left untreated, can become very serious and even life-threatening called Stevens-Johnson Syndrome (SJS). However, around 10% of people taking lamotrigine develop a benign rash. Slower and smaller dose changes decrease the risk of developing a rash. It is important to monitor yourself for a rash, especially around dose changes, and see your doctor if one occurs. Most times, the rash disappears once the medication is discontinued.

Antipsychotics

These medications are used at higher doses to treat schizophrenia, severe bipolar disorders, and other psychoses. They are increasingly used at lower doses, in combination with an antidepressant, to manage anxiety and unipolar depression. The antipsychotics included here are considered "atypical" antipsychotics, as compared with the first generation of antipsychotic medications, e.g., Haldol.

Quetiapine (Seroquel)

TYPE	USED FOR
atypical antipsychotic, mood stabilizer	schizophrenia[US,CA]
	acute mania[US,CA]
	maintenance therapy in bipolar disorder[US]
ACTS ON	bipolar depression[US,CA]
dopamine, serotonin	depression[US,CA]
	other psychosis

Typically used at higher doses to address psychosis, at lower doses, it is often used to help with overall mood stability, aggression, anxiety and insomnia. It can help prevent nightmares in PTSD. Unlike many sedatives and hypnotics, it is not addictive, so it can be used long term if needed. It can be associated with metabolic syndrome (e.g., weight gain, increased cholesterol, diabetes), especially at higher doses. Initial metabolic testing and periodic monitoring are warranted. Immediate and extended-release formulations are available.

Antipsychotics

Risperidone (Risperdal)

TYPE
atypical antipsychotic, mood stabilizer

ACTS ON
dopamine, serotonin, norepinephrine

USED FOR
schizophrenia[US,CA]
acute mania[US,CA]
maintenance therapy in bipolar disorder[US]
bipolar depression
impulse control disorders

Like quetiapine, it is used at higher doses for psychosis and lower doses for overall mood stability, aggression, and agitation. It is less sedating than quetiapine. Unlike many sedatives and hypnotics, it is not addictive, so it can be used long term if needed.

Metabolic syndrome is again a concern, so initial metabolic testing and periodic monitoring are warranted. Below 6mg, most people experience less weight gain on risperidone than quetiapine or olanzapine. Above 6mg, side effects commonly seen with typical antipsychotics can occur, e.g., parkinsonism. It can cause elevated prolactin levels in some people, possibly causing breast tenderness and lactation. Long term, increased prolactin can cause osteoporosis, so it is important to report these symptoms to your doctor.

Olanzapine (Zyprexa)

TYPE
atypical antipsychotic, mood stabilizer

ACTS ON
dopamine, serotonin

USED FOR
schizophrenia[US,CA]
acute mania[US,CA]
maintenance therapy in bipolar disorder[US,CA]
bipolar depression[US†]
depression[US†]
other psychosis
impulse control disorders
borderline personality disorder

Like risperidone, it is used at higher doses for psychosis and lower doses for overall mood stability, anxiety, aggression, and agitation. It is also often used to augment other medications when treating unipolar or bipolar depression. It can be used long term if needed. It is fairly sedating. Many people experience significant weight gain and metabolic syndrome. Initial metabolic testing and periodic monitoring are warranted.

Lurasidone (Latuda)

TYPE
atypical antipsychotic

ACTS ON
dopamine, serotonin

USED FOR
schizophrenia[US,CA]
bipolar depression[US,CA]
acute mania
maintenance therapy in bipolar disorder
depression
other psychosis
impulse control disorders

Lurasidone is one of the better-tolerated antipsychotics, used for similar purposes. It does not usually cause weight gain over the long term, though it is often somewhat sedating. Unlike some of the other medications, it can be taken once a day but needs to be taken with at least 350 calories of food.

Aripiprazole (Abilify)

TYPE
atypical antipsychotic, mood stabilizer

ACTS ON
dopamine, serotonin

USED FOR
schizophrenia[US,CA]
acute mania[US]
maintenance therapy in bipolar disorder[US]
depression[US]
bipolar depression
other psychosis
impulse control disorders

Aripiprazole is not as frequently associated with either weight gain or sedation. At lower doses (1-5mg), it is often used to augment antidepressants ("augment with Abilify!" proclaims the advertising). Some people find it activating. This can help with symptoms of depression like anhedonia and fatigue. It also treats cognitive symptoms. Watch for feelings of inner motor restlessness. A successor medication, brexpiprazole (Rexulti) is also now available.

Stimulants and Related

This section includes medications for ADHD. These medications are also used to augment antidepressants to improve concentration, fatigue, and inattention due to other causes like depression.

The most common agents are stimulants based on either amphetamine or methylphenidate. Some non-stimulant medications in this category are also available that don't have the same abuse potential.

Amphetamine (Dexedrine, Adderall, Vyvanse)

TYPE
stimulant

ACTS ON
dopamine, norepinephrine

USED FOR
ADHD[US]
narcolepsy[US†,CA†]
binge eating disorder[US†,CA†]
treatment-resistant depression

Amphetamine-based psychostimulants are primarily used to treat ADHD, and often as an augmenting agent to improve cognitive symptoms of depression. Lisdexamfetamine (Vyvanse) is the only one approved for binge eating disorder.

Because they use different delivery mechanisms, the length of time they work varies. Overall, they start working quickly. Their effect peaks within an hour or two, then gradually tails off. For example:

- Dexedrine (one peak, lasts ~4h)
- Dexedrine spansules (one peak, lasts ~6-8h)
- Adderall XR (one peak, lasts ~12h)
- Vyvanse (one peak, then fairly level, lasts ~13-14h)

Methylphenidate (Ritalin, Concerta, Aptensio)

TYPE
stimulant

ACTS ON
dopamine, norepinephrine

USED FOR
ADHD[US,CA]
narcolepsy[US†,CA†]
treatment-resistant depression

The other main psychostimulant medications are those made of methylphenidate. As with the amphetamine-based medications, a variety of delivery mechanisms are used which provide different durations and patterns of effect. Most start working quickly, their effect peaking within an hour or two, and then gradually tail off. Some have a second peak, a few hours after the first, as if you'd taken a second dose. For example:

- Ritalin (one peak, lasts ~3-4h)
- Ritalin LA (two peaks, lasts ~6-8h)
- Concerta (one peak, lasts ~12h)
- Aptensio/Biphentin (two peaks, lasts ~10-12h)

Atomoxetine (Strattera)

TYPE
selective norepinephrine reuptake inhibitor

USED FOR
ADHD[US,CA]
treatment-resistant depression

ACTS ON
norepinephrine, dopamine

Atomoxetine is a non-stimulant medication for the treatment of ADHD, which does not have abuse potential like the amphetamine- and methylphenidate-based medications. Those with bipolar disorders should watch for the possible development of a hypomanic or manic episode.

Other Stimulants and Related

Several other medications are commonly used for symptoms of ADHD, fatigue, concentration, etc. Guanfacine (Intuniv) is a blood pressure medication that has also been approved for ADHD. Like atomoxetine, it also has no known abuse potential. Clonidine is another blood pressure medication with similar properties. Modafinil (Alertec), another low-abuse alternative to stimulants, is approved to treat excessive sleepiness in narcolepsy, shift workers, sleep apnea, and fatigue due to other physical illness. It also helps improve attention in ADHD and fatigue. The antidepressant bupropion (Wellbutrin) can also provide some help for these symptoms.

Notes

Chapter 2. What Is Mental Illness?

1. Courtesy the Mayo Clinic
   ↪ https://www.mayoclinic.org

2. Two separate large studies in the USA provided a good picture of the risk of mental illness and which mental illnesses are more likely to occur together.
   Kessler RC, Chiu WT, Demler O, Walters EE. "Prevalence, Severity, and Comorbidity of 12-Month DSM-IV Disorders in the National Comorbidity Survey Replication." *Archives of General Psychiatry.* 2005;62(6):617–627.
   ↪ https://doi.org/10.1001/archpsyc.62.6.617
   Hasin DS, Goodwin RD, Stinson FS, Grant BF. "Epidemiology of Major Depressive Disorder: Results From the National Epidemiologic Survey on Alcoholism and Related Conditions." *Archives of General Psychiatry.* 2005;62(10):1097–1106.
   ↪ https://doi.org/10.1001/archpsyc.62.10.1097

3. Thanks to DJ Jaffe for highlighting those examples. The data on ADHD rates were reported in a New York Times article, based on a study by the Centers for Disease Control. The rate for teenage girls was about half that of boys, and half the boys diagnosed were on ADHD medications. The second example was based on databases of hospital discharges over ten years in both the USA and the UK.
   Schwarz A, Cohen S. "More Diagnoses of Hyperactivity in New Centers for Disease Control Data." *New York Times.* April 1, 2013.
   ↪ https://mhnav.com/r/nytdxhyp
   James A, Hoang U, Seagroatt V, Clacey J, et al. "A Comparison of American and English Hospital Discharge Rates for Pediatric Bipolar Disorder, 2000 to 2010," *Journal of the American Academy of Child & Adolescent Psychiatry.* 2014;53(6):614–24.
   ↪ https://doi.org/10.1016/j.jaac.2014.02.008

4. One reliable source of data is the annual U.S. National Survey on Drug Use and Health (NSDUH). This survey is undertaken by the Substance Abuse and Men-

tal Health Services Administration (SAMHSA). It collects data from about 68,000 people, taking into account gender, age, race, geography, income, insurance, and overall health.

The 2016 survey classified 18.3% of respondents as having a mental illness in the past year and 4.2% having a severe mental illness. The full reports and data are available.

↪ https://www.samhsa.gov/data/population-data-nsduh/

Chapter 4. The Mental Health System

1. Programs for severe mental illness also have significant problems, and don't get all the resources they need—far from it.

Arguably, the system wastes a sizeable chunk of mental health funds on people who don't need help or won't benefit. These funds could be better spent on those with greater need. This is a large and important topic in its own right but beyond the scope of this book. For some incredible and shocking insights into these issues in the American system, we would recommend the book *Insane Consequences* by DJ Jaffe.

↪ https://mentalillnesspolicy.org/insane-consequences.html

2. A variety of studies have looked at this question, using surveys of family doctors, as well as by examining administrative (i.e. billing) data, across various geographic areas. The 20% figure +/- 5% comes up frequently. A representative example of this is a paper describing a family doctor survey done in Quebec.

Fleury MJ, Farand L, Aube D, Imboua A. "Management of mental health problems by general practitioners in Quebec." *Canadian Family Physician.* 2012;58:e732–8.

↪ http://www.cfp.ca/content/cfp/58/12/e732.full.pdf

Chapter 5. Taking an Active Role

1. In public health systems, this raises ethical and policy questions. Does the ability to pay provide someone with a better level of essential treatment? As with many other aspects of healthcare, the answer appears to be yes.

Alter DA, Iron K, Austin P, Naylor D. "Socioeconomic Status, Service Patterns, and Perceptions of Care Among Survivors of Acute Myocardial Infarction in Canada." *Journal of the American Medical Association.* 2004;291(9):1100–1107.

↪ https://doi.org/10.1001/jama.291.9.1100

2. These articles give a bit of context around the rise of patient navigation. They emphasize that the demand has increased because the healthcare system has become more complex. The first two are from news outlets in Canada. The last, an opinion piece by a US doctor, notes that there at least, some navigators help patients with their complex medical bills.

Grant K. "Patients resort to paying consultants to help navigate Canada's Byzantine health-care system.". *The Globe & Mail.* April 14, 2017.

↪ https://mhnav.com/r/gmptnavs

CTVNews.ca staff, "Private patient advocates help out—for a price." *CTV News.* Jun 19, 2017.
↪ https://mhnav.com/r/ctvppadv

Kirsch M. "The rise of patient navigators is a sign that medical billing needs to be reformed." via *KevinMD.* Nov 12, 2017.
↪ https://mhnav.com/r/navbilkm

Chapter 6. Get Prepared

1. You can find many templates for safety plans online. Here's one from the National Suicide Prevention Lifeline in the USA:
↪ https://mhnav.com/r/safeplan

Chapter 7. Family and Friends

1. One book that we'd highly recommend is *Lost Marbles: Insights into My Life with Depression and Bipolar* by Natasha Tracy (2016). She's a mental health advocate who has a severe bipolar disorder. Her well-written and well-researched book paints a vivid picture of a variety of mental health symptoms. More information can be found on her website.
↪ http://natashatracy.com

Other recommended authors are Barbara Lipska (*The Neuroscientist Who Lost Her Mind*), Susannah Calahan (*Brain on Fire*), Kay Redfield Jamison (*An Unquiet Mind*), Romeo Dallaire (*Waiting for First Light*), Elizabeth Wurtzel (*Prozac Nation*), Terri Cheney (*Manic: A Memoir*), Mary Karr (*Lit*), and Susanna Kaysen (*Girl Interrupted*).

If you enjoy humour intertwined with accurate portrayals of mental illness, look for books by Jenny Lawson (*Furiously Happy*), Allie Brosh (*Hyperbole and a Half*), and Carrie Fisher (*Wishful Drinking*).

Not first-person, but books by Oliver Sacks (*The Man Who Mistook His Wife For a Hat*) will give you piercing insight into a range of psychiatric and neurological conditions.

Chapter 8. Working With Your Family Doctor

1. In the USA, the main gatekeeper is usually not doctors, but insurance companies. They decide if tests will be paid for or not.

Self-referral for diagnostic tests or other expensive services in the USA results in overuse of services, though many of the costs are born by those who purchase these services. Doctors more worried about liability will also order more unnecessary tests, known as *defensive (or CYA) medicine.*

Hendee WR, Becker GJ, Borgstede JP, Bosma J, et al. "Addressing Overutilization in Medical Imaging." *Radiology.* 2010;257(1):240-245.
↪ https://doi.org/10.1148/radiol.10100063

The *Choosing Wisely* initiative helps patients and doctors identify and reduce the use of unnecessary testing.
↪ http://choosingwisely.org

2. Doctor burnout is a growing problem. It has received more attention lately, at least within the medical community. In the USA, much of this stems from a loss of autonomy and greater administrative demands as healthcare organizations grow. For example, great effort is put into meeting new documentation requirements that add little to clinical care but are needed for billing and compliance with meaningful use legislation.

The work that doctors do is stressful enough. The medical culture makes it worse. There is intense competition to both enter and then succeed in medicine. Needing help is seen as a weakness and can, at times, have damaging career consequences. With few perceived options but easy access to pharmaceuticals to self-medicate, addiction and suicide are common. Numbers vary, but suicide rates are roughly 2-3x the general population.

For those interested, a good starting point is the online doctor community KevinMD.
↪ https://kevinmd.com

Pamela Wible is the most visible advocate for addressing doctor suicide. Her blog and TED talk are good introductions.
↪ https://idealmedicalcare.org

3. Yes, it's a real thing. If you're interested in exploring what can happens when celebrity culture meets health advice, we'd highly recommend health science expert Timothy Caulfield's 2015 book, *Is Gwyneth Paltrow Wrong About Everything? When Celebrity Culture and Science Clash*.

4. Unfortunately, there is a large and varied body of research correlating mental illness (even, e.g., mild major depressive disorder) with poor physical health. Some of this work looks at health outcomes, e.g. five-year survival rate after a cardiac event is lower for those with mental illness. Patients with mental illness are less likely to follow their treatment plan, likely contributing to this statistic. Other studies look at how often particular interventions are offered and find that people with mental illness are less likely to undergo a procedure like cardiac catheterization after a heart attack. Studies have found that the rates of certain common lab tests for physical health conditions can be lower in those with mental illness. Some of these studies focus on severe mental illness while others are more broad. Many use very large healthcare databases, while others use specific patient demographics (e.g. patients in Veterans hospitals).

Determining the exact reasons why patients with mental illness receive poorer physical health treatment is decidedly tricky. There are many potential confounding variables. Nevertheless, the data is pretty strong across a wide range of medical environments. Stigma among many healthcare providers against those with mental illness likely plays a role.

Of the hundreds of papers available, we've included a very small selection of papers addressing these topics.

Druss BG, Bradford DW, Rosenheck RA, Radford MJ, Krumholz HM. "Mental disorders and use of cardiovascular procedures after myocardial infarction." *Journal of the American Medical Association.* 2000;283(4):506-511.
↳ https://doi.org/10.1001/jama.283.4.506

Druss BG, Bradford DW, Rosenheck RA, Radford MJ, Krumholz HM. "Quality of Medical Care and Excess Mortality in Older Patients With Mental Disorders." *Archives of General Psychiatry.* 2001;58(6):565-572.
↳ https://doi.org/10.1001/archpsyc.58.6.565

Frayne SM, Halanych JH, Miller DR, Wang F, et al. "Disparities in Diabetes Care: Impact of Mental Illness." *Archives of Internal Medicine.* 2005;165(22):2631-2638.
↳ https://doi.org/10.1001/archinte.165.22.2631

Mitchell AJ, Malone D, Doebbeling CC. "Quality of medical care for people with and without comorbid mental illness and substance misuse: systematic review of comparative studies." *British Journal of Psychiatry.* 2009;194(6):491-499.
↳ https://doi.org/10.1192/bjp.bp.107.045732

Jones S, Howard L, Thornicroft G. "'Diagnostic overshadowing': worse physical health care for people with mental illness." *Acta Psychiatrica Scandinavia.* 2008;118(3):169-171.
↳ https://doi.org/10.1111/j.1600-0447.2008.01211.x

Chapter 10. Working the Waiting List

1. Every clinic or service has their own process. Some may randomly assign doctors to patients. Some may pick the next doctor available. Still others may try to match the patient's needs outlined in the referral information with the doctor who they think would be the best fit.

2. One of the most popular doctor rating sites in Canada and the USA is RateMDs. Think of it as Yelp! or TripAdvisor for doctors.
↳ https://www.ratemds.com

Chapter 12. Difficult Encounters

1. Before someone can practice as a fully-licensed specialist, they need to successfully complete certain training, be observed and evaluated by supervising specialists, and pass exams. When doctors move from other countries, their training is assessed. Often, they need to write the same exams, redo some or all of their residency training, and/or practice under someone's supervision for a time to demonstrate competency. Only then are they fully qualified to practice independently.

In this case, the doctor hadn't completed one or more of those steps. Their license to practice medicine, in Alberta, was classified as "Provisional Register Conditional Non-specialist Defined Practice." That is for "non-specialist physicians in a specialty discipline, who are in the process of qualifying for the General Register but do not yet meet the full criteria."

We recently checked, and that particular doctor had just fully qualified as meeting national standards, and now had a "full" license to practice as a psychiatrist. They'd held the same conditional license for *six years*. That's longer than doctors spend in training after medical school to become psychiatrists in the first place.

2. After all, why say "dysthymia" when you could say "persistent depressive disorder, severe, late-onset, with anxious distress (moderate-severe), without psychotic features, with intermittent major depressive episodes, without current episode, in partial remission?"

Chapter 13. Paging Dr. Google

1. To learn more, visit the Stop Predatory Journals website.
   ↪ https://predatoryjournals.com

2. This blog post by one doctor provides extra guidance about sharing what you've found.
   Njiaju UO. "Do's and don'ts for patients who consult Dr. Google." via *KevinMD*. Oct 22, 2017.
   ↪ https://mhnav.com/r/ptgoogkm

Chapter 16. So Many Choices!

1. We're not able to include all possible interventions and treatments. We excluded those predominantly used in severe mental illnesses markedly affecting the ability to meaningfully participate in care decisions. We prioritized common evidence-based interventions for mental disorders that readers of this book would most often experience.

We excluded countless medications, supplements, forms of psychotherapy, etc. Many complementary and alternative medical interventions, including acupuncture, relaxation therapies, massage, and light therapy, are not included. Don't interpret the omission of any particular treatment here as a value judgment or claim that it can't help you.

Chapter 18. Physical Illness

1. Qato DM, Ozenberger K, Olfson M. "Prevalence of Prescription Medications With Depression as a Potential Adverse Effect Among Adults in the United States." *Journal of the American Medical Association*. 2018;319(22):2289–2298.
   ↪ https://doi.org/10.1001/jama.2018.6741

The study authors also analyzed their data to remove any psychotropic medications from the list. They still found a similar result. Taking multiple medications with depression as a side effect increased the risk of developing depression. We don't know whether the medications were the direct cause of the study participants' depressions. The illnesses for which these medications were taken could play a part. The psychosocial factors (e.g. disability, financial strain) they were experiencing could also have an effect.

2. This article from the Canadian Mental Health Association provides a good overview of the complex interactions and consequences of comorbid physical and mental illness:

↳ https://mhnav.com/r/cmhamhpc

The article, as well as some of the examples from it we're using here, represent very general and high-level conclusions. They omit many details and caveats contained in the original studies they refer to.

3. Diagnostic overshadowing was a term originally used when referring to patients with mental retardation. It has since been applied to patients with a full range of mental illnesses.

Mason J, Scior K. " 'Diagnostic Overshadowing' Amongst Clinicians Working with People with Intellectual Disabilities in the UK." *Journal of Applied Research in Intellectual Disabilities.* 2004;17(2):85-90.

↳ https://doi.org/10.1111/j.1360-2322.2004.00184.x

Jones S, Howard L, Thornicroft G. " 'Diagnostic overshadowing': worse physical health care for people with mental illness." *Acta Psychiatrica Scandinavica.* 2008;118(3):169-171.

↳ https://doi.org/10.1111/j.1600-0447.2008.01211.x

Thornicroft G, Rose D, Kassam A. "Discrimination in health care against people with mental illness." *International Review of Psychiatry.* 2007;19(2):113-22.

↳ https://doi.org/10.1080/09540260701278937

Chapter 19. Lab Investigations

1. If and how lab results are shared varies by jurisdiction and organization. Some of the variation is due to logistics (e.g., hooking everything up), maintenance costs, and privacy concerns. and who is going to pay to maintain that service. Some of this is concerns over privacy rights. For example, in Alberta, there is a central database called NetCare for all lab results. It lets doctors look up results online. The catch is that not every doctor can use NetCare (especially those in smaller offices), due to very rigid privacy safeguards.

2. Practice guidelines can be either vague ("for high-risk patients") or altogether silent around who should be screened or monitored. A group in the Netherlands recently proposed a pragmatic set of criteria as a starting point to help fill this gap.

Simoons M, Seldenrijk A, Mulder H, Birkenhager T, et al. "Limited Evidence for Risk Factors for Proarrthymia and Sudden Cardiac Death in Patients Using Antidepressants: Dutch Consensus on ECG Monitoring." *Drug Safety.* 2018;41(7):655-664.

↳ https://doi.org/10.1007/s40264-018-0649-z

Chapter 20. Lifestyle Factors

1. The CDC in the United States, via The National Health and Nutrition Examination Survey, collected blood and urine samples to measure a wide variety of nutrients and other biochemical indicators.
    ↪ https://www.cdc.gov/nutritionreport/

2. One book that we continue to recommend is *Becoming Vegan* by dieticians Brenda Davis and Vesanto Melina. It provides high-quality and extensive information on dietary sources of nutrients. It comprehensively discusses each nutrient, its role in our body, the amount in many different foods, and how deficiency affects us. Carnivores will likely skip past the advocacy chapter. Note that animal products are included "for comparison purposes." There are now two versions, an "Express" edition and a 600+ page "Comprehensive" edition.
    ↪ https://becomingvegan.ca

3. Suggestions for improving your sleep hygiene can be easily found online. Here's one list from the sleep information site Tuck.com:
    ↪ https://www.tuck.com/sleep-hygiene/

4. This data was from the 2015 Canadian Tobacco Alcohol and Drugs Survey (CTADS). It was collected through telephone interviews of 15,000+ Canadians ages 15 years and older. Of note, those aged 15–24 were far more likely to be current users of cannabis rather than tobacco.
    ↪ https://mhnav.com/r/canatads

    In the United States, the National Survey on Drug Use and Health, directed by SAMHSA, provides detailed information, broken down across various demographic factors. In the 2016 survey, overall cannabis use was 13.7%, peaking at 32.5% in the 18–25 age group. Interestingly, though cannabis use in the USA and Canada were close (13.7% versus 12.3%), tobacco use was much higher in the USA (overall 25% versus 13%).
    ↪ https://mhnav.com/r/usansduh

    Both Canadian and US numbers refer to the percentage of current users. They don't say anything about the frequency or quantity of use.

    For a more international perspective, the 2017 World Drug Report by the United Nations Office on Drugs and Crime is a good source.
    ↪ https://www.unodc.org/wdr2017/

5. These guidelines were developed by the Canadian Research Initiative in Substance Misuse (CRISM). CAMH has two short brochures summarizing the guidelines, one for the public and one for health professionals. Details on the methodology and sources of data behind the recommendations are also available.
    ↪ https://mhnav.com/r/lrcugpub
    ↪ https://mhnav.com/r/lrcugpro
    ↪ https://doi.org/10.2105/AJPH.2017.303818

6. Research on hallucinogens started in the 1950's and early 1960's, but came to an abrupt halt in the mid-1960's when LSD and other psychedelics were criminalized. There has been a resurgence of research since the late 1990's. Broadly, the use

of some psychedelics during specialized psychotherapy sessions may shorten the overall course of therapy. For those who are curious, a good starting point is the 2018 book by Michael Pollan, *How to Change Your Mind: What the New Science of Psychedelics Teaches Us About Consciousness, Dying, Addiction, Depression, and Transcendence*.

Chapter 21. Vitamins and Supplements

1. Kessler RC, Soukup J, Davis RB, Foster DF, et al. "The Use of Complementary and Alternative Therapies to Treat Anxiety and Depression in the United States." *American Journal of Psychiatry*. 2001;158(2):289-294.
   ↪ https://doi.org/10.1176/appi.ajp.158.2.289

2. Eisenberg DM, Davis RB, Ettner SL, Appel S, et al. "Trends in Alternative Medicine Use in the United States, 1990-1997: Results of a Follow-up National Survey." *Journal of the American Medical Association*. 1998;280(18):1569–1575.
   ↪ https://doi.org/10.1001/jama.280.18.1569

3. Both Health Canada and the National Institutes of Health in the USA publish guidelines on nutrient intake. The main Office of Dietary Supplements website also publishes many useful fact sheets on individual nutrients, including what the nutrient does, the effects of deficiency, possible interactions, best food sources, and more. It also provides information on common supplements.
   ↪ https://mhnav.com/r/hcadrfik
   ↪ https://mhnav.com/r/nihdrfik
   ↪ https://ods.od.nih.gov

4. Shaw KA, Turner J, Del Mar C. "Tryptophan and 5-Hydroxytryptophan for depression." *Cochrane Database of Systematic Reviews*. 2002(1).
   ↪ https://doi.org/10.1002/14651858.CD003198

5. Sarris J, Murphy J, Mischoulon D, Papkostas GI, et al. "Adjunctive Nutraceuticals for Depression: A Systematic Review and Meta-Analyses." *American Journal of Psychiatry*. 2016;173(6):575-587.
   ↪ https://doi.org/10.1176/appi.ajp.2016.15091228

6. A good recent review examined the mixed results of Omega-3 in a range of mental health conditions. Later commentary discussed the difficulty trying to draw firm conclusions from existing research.
   Bozzatello P, Brignolo E, De Grandi E, Bellino S. "Supplementation with Omega-3 Fatty Acids in Psychiatric Disorders: A Review of Literature Data." *Journal of Clinical Medicine*. 2016;5(8),67.
   ↪ https://doi.org/10.3390/jcm5080067
   Berger G. "Comments on Bozzatello et al. Supplementation with Omega-3 Fatty Acids in Psychiatric Disorders: A Review of Literature Data." *Journal of Clinical Medicine*. 2016;5(8),69.
   ↪ https://doi.org/10.3390/jcm5080069

7. Sateia MJ, Buysse DJ, Krystal AD, Neubauer DN, Heald JL. "Clinical Practice Guideline for the Pharmacologic Treatment of Chronic Insomnia in Adults: An American Academy of Sleep Medicine Clinical Practice Guideline." *Journal of Clinical Sleep Medicine.* 2017;13(2):307-349.

↪ https://doi.org/10.5664/jcsm.6470

8. Saeed M, Naveed M, Arif M, Kakar MU, et al. "Green tea (Camellia sinensis) and l-theanine: Medicinal values and beneficial applications in humans—A comprehensive review." *Biomedicine & Pharmacotherapy.* 2017;95:1260-1275.

↪ https://doi.org/10.1016/j.biopha.2017.09.024

9. Kim H, McGrath B, Silverstone PH. "A review of the possible relevance of inositol and the phosphatidylinositol second messenger system (PI-cycle) to psychiatric disorders—Focus on magnetic resonance spectroscopy (MRS) studies." *Human Psychopharmacology: Clinical & Experimental.* 2005;20(5):309-326.

↪ https://doi.org/10.1002/hup.693

10. Poly C, Massaro JM, Seshadri S, Wolf PA, et al. "The relation of dietary choline to cognitive performance and white-matter hyperintensity in the Framingham Offspring Cohort." *American Journal of Clinical Nutrition.* 2011;94(6):1584-1591.

↪ https://doi.org/10.3945/ajcn.110.008938

11. Jongkees BJ, Hommel B, Kuhn S, Colzato LS. "Effect of tyrosine supplementation on clinical and healthy populations under stress or cognitive demands—A review." *Journal of Psychiatric Research.* 2015;70:50-57.

↪ https://doi.org/10.1016/j.jpsychires.2015.08.014

12. UHND staff. "2 Natural Antidepressants Found to Be as Effective as Prozac." *University Health News Daily.* Nov 24, 2017.

↪ https://mhnav.com/r/uhnadnat

13. Sarris J, Panossian A, Schweitzer I, Stough C, Scholey A. "Herbal medicine for depression, anxiety and insomnia: A review of psychopharmacology and clinical evidence." *European Neuropsychopharmacology.* 2011;21(12):841-860.

↪ https://doi.org/10.1016/j.euroneuro.2011.04.002

14. Apaydin EA, Maher AR, Shanman R, Booth MS, et al. "A systematic review of St. John's wort for major depressive disorder." *Systematic Reviews.* 2016;5(1):148-172.

↪ https://doi.org/10.1186/s13643-016-0325-2

15. Saeed SA, Bloch RM, Antonacci DJ. "Herbal and Dietary Supplements for Treatment of Anxiety Disorders." *American Family Physician.* 2007;76(4):549-556.

↪ https://www.aafp.org/afp/2007/0815/p549.html

16. Sarris J, Panossian A, Schweitzer I, Stough C, Scholey A. "Herbal medicine for depression, anxiety and insomnia: A review of psychopharmacology and clinical evidence." *European Neuropsychopharmacology.* 2011;21(12):841-860.

↪ https://doi.org/10.1016/j.euroneuro.2011.04.002

17. This extreme story illustrates how few safeguards are present in the natural health system around manufacturing, evidence, and sales practices. We'd encourage you to seek out the 2003 e-book "Pig Pills Inc: The Anatomy of an Academic and Alternative Health Fraud" by Terry Polevoy MD, Ron Reinhold, and Marvin Ross. More information can be found at:
↪ http://pigpills.com

18. If you're interested, you can find online tools to check medication and supplement interactions on sites like rxlist.com and drugs.com. As always, only your healthcare providers can interpret how these might apply to you. You'll find more information about this in the *Antidepressants* chapter, under the heading Metabolism and Interactions.

Chapter 22. Talk Therapy

1. The Canadian Network for Mood and Anxiety Treatments publish a variety of treatment guidelines, as well as other research.
↪ https://canmat.org

Chapter 23. Finding a Therapist

1. Providers may understand the value of many treatments, yet only *offer* a few. This is very common. A psychiatrist might agree that medications and psychotherapy would be helpful but only offer medication management. They would recommend that patients see someone else for psychotherapy.

Chapter 24. The Role of Medications

1. The formal name for this measure is the *number needed to treat (NNT)*. It's a frequently used measure of effectiveness in evidence-based medicine. The corresponding measure for treatment safety is the *number needed to harm (NNH)*. A group of doctors have scoured studies to collect NNT data on a wide range of medical conditions and interventions.
↪ https://thennt.com

Their site is unfortunately short on data surrounding psychiatric treatments (and a few other areas) but is a great resource to put specific NNT data in context (e.g., compare your treatments with others). Data on specific treatments for specific conditions, mental health and otherwise, can easily be found by searching Cochrane reviews and Google Scholar.

Chapter 25. Antidepressants

1. Kennedy SH, Lam RW, McIntyre RS, Tourjman SV, et al. "Canadian Network for Mood and Anxiety Treatments (CANMAT) 2016 clinical guidelines for the

management of adults with major depressive disorder: Section 3. Pharmacological Treatments." *Canadian Journal of Psychiatry.* 2016;61(9):540-560.
↪ https://doi.org/10.1177/0706743716659417

2. Volpi-Abadie J, Kaye AM, Kaye AD. "Serotonin syndrome". *The Ochsner Journal.* 2013;13(4):533–40.
↪ https://www.ncbi.nlm.nih.gov/pmc/articles/PMC3865832/

3. Except for overdose, serotonin syndrome is virtually always a result of combining two or more serotonergic medications or nutraceuticals. Yet, some medications remain in the body for days or weeks after they've been stopped (e.g. fluoxetine). While you may be on only one serotonergic medication now, make sure doctors know if you've recently stopped another.

Serotonin syndrome can also be brought on by adding medications or nutraceuticals that aren't themselves serotonergic! As we mentioned previously, some medications affect the liver pathways that break down medications and remove them from your system. That could result in toxic levels of a serotonergic medication, which could lead to serotonin syndrome. However, serotonin syndrome is very rare.

Chapter 26. Other Medications

1. Healthcare workers refer to medications you take only when needed (rather than on a regular schedule) as *p.r.n.* medications. This is from *pro re nata*, the Latin translation of "when needed." This is the extent of your Latin lessons!

2. Dr. Heather Ashton maintains a very useful website about benzodiazepines, covering a range of topics. It includes step-by-step protocols to gradually reduce and stop benzodiazepines. The first steps are converting other benzodiazepines to their equivalent dose of diazepam. The long half-life of diazepam helps minimize withdrawal as it is reduced. You can find more information at:
↪ https://benzo.org.uk

Chapter 27. Medication Side Effects

1. Have you ever seen studies that compare a medication to placebo? They show that people who take the actual medication report side effects. Bizarrely, those given the placebo also report side effects! It's called the *nocebo* effect. It reflects peoples' expectations and fears around medications.

Sometimes the nocebo effect can be quite significant. Consider a study used to get FDA approval of the antidepressant escitalopram to treat generalized anxiety disorder. It showed that 24% of people taking the medication developed headaches. But, 17% of the people taking a placebo also reported developing headaches. The actual difference of 7% is far more modest.
↪ https://mhnav.com/r/fdaescit

2. Physician practice varies when treating side effects. Keep in mind there are usually multiple ways to address any issue.

Dording CM, Mischoulon D, Petersen TJ, Kornbluh R, et al. "The Pharmacologic Management of SSRI-Induced Side Effects: A Survey of Psychiatrists." *Annals of Clinical Psychiatry.* 2002;14(3):143-147.
↪ https://doi.org/10.3109/10401230209147450

Goldberg JF, Ernst CL. *Managing the Side Effects of Psychotropic Medications.* American Psychiatric Publishing, 2012.

3. Many general articles about side effects (such as the Dording et al. article cited in the previous section) include extensive information on sexual side effects in particular. Two additional reports are noted here.

Taylor MJ, Rudkin L, Bullemor-Day P, Lubin J, et al. "Strategies for managing sexual dysfunction induced by antidepressant medication." *Cochrane Database of Systematic Reviews.* 2013(5).
↪ https://doi.org/10.1002/14651858.CD003382.pub3

Nurnberg HG, Hensley PL, Gelenberg AJ, Fava M, et al. "Treatment of Antidepressant-Associated Sexual Dysfunction With Sildenafil: A Randomized Controlled Trial." *Journal of the American Medical Association.* 2003;289(1):56-64.
↪ https://doi.org/10.1001/jama.289.1.56

4. Holbrook AM, Crowther R, Lotter A, Cheng C, King D. "The diagnosis and management of insomnia in clinical practice: a practical evidence-based approach." *Canadian Medical Association Journal.* 2000;162(2):216-210.
↪ http://www.cmaj.ca/content/162/2/216

5. Lieberman JA. "Managing anticholinergic side effects." *Primary Care Companion to the Journal of Clinical Psychiatry.* 2004;6(2):20-23.
↪ https://www.ncbi.nlm.nih.gov/pmc/articles/PMC487008/

6. Zeisel SH, da Costa KA. "Choline: an essential nutrient for public health" *Nutrition Reviews.* 2009;67(11):615-623.
↪ https://www.ncbi.nlm.nih.gov/pmc/articles/PMC2782876/

Chapter 28. Evolving Your Medication Regime

1. Why applesauce but not chocolate pudding? It turns out applesauce has the correct pH to maintain the extended-release properties of this specific medication, while chocolate pudding will ruin them. And yes, there's a study to back it up. It was done because some elderly patients had difficulty swallowing the capsule; applesauce and chocolate pudding are readily available in most elder care facilities.

Wells KA, Losin WG. "In vitro stability, potency, and dissolution of duloxetine enteric-coated pellets after exposure to applesauce, apple juice, and chocolate pudding." *Clinical Therapeutics.* 2008;30(7):1300-1308.
↪ https://doi.org/10.1016/S0149-2918(08)80054-9

2. The Centers for Disease Control and Prevention has some good information on birth defects, including data for the United States.
↪ https://www.cdc.gov/ncbddd/birthdefects/data.html

3. Andres RL, Day MC. "Perinatal complications associated with maternal tobacco use." *Seminars in Neonatology*. 2000;5(3):231–241.
↪ https://doi.org/10.1053/siny.2000.0025

4. A small study by Motherisk investigated the fear of psychotropic medications in pregnancy, the consequences of abruptly stopping medications, and the role that counselling can play in helping women evaluate the risks and benefits.
↪ https://www.ncbi.nlm.nih.gov/pmc/articles/PMC1408034

5. OTIS, the Organization of Teratology Information Specialists (teratology is the study of congenital abnormalities) carries out numerous research studies and has published a great deal of information on medication in pregnancy on their website. Their fact sheets are particularly useful.
↪ https://mothertobaby.org

Chapter 29. Looking Ahead

1. These mental health navigation services usually start by reviewing your case and connecting you with the right mental health provider. Some are part of existing services that connect people with a range of medical specialists.
↪ https://bestdoctors.com

Others are dedicated entirely to mental health care navigation, like this small company in California:
↪ https://merrittmentalhealth.com

Index

5-HTP, 145

Abilify, *see* aripiprazole
absorption, 128, 134, 187
Acceptance and Commitment Therapy, *see* ACT
ACT, 236
Adams, Douglas, ix
Adderall, *see* amphetamine
addiction, 46, 142, 200
ADHD, 12, 19, 186, 208, 256
    medications, 199
adrenaline, 130, 137, 154
akathisia, 208
alcohol, 138–139, 190
Alertec, *see* modafinil
alprazolam, 248
amantadine, 205
Ambien, *see* zolpidem
amitriptyline, 246
amphetamine, 257
Anafranil, *see* clomipramine
anger, *see* irritability
anorexia nervosa, 16, 133
anosognosia, 13
anti-psychiatry, 83, 174
anticholinergic, 147, 207–209
antidepressants, 177–190
antipsychotics, 197–198
    cognitive problems, 208

anxiety, 73
    internet, 81
    interviews, 68
    medication, 168, 177, 182, 185, 191, 202
    risk, 121, 123, 137, 138, 140
    scales, 57
    side effect, 123
    treatment, 19, 24, 128, 130, 135, 143, 148, 154, 175, 233
    types, 74
anxiolytics, *see* sedatives
appointments, 41–42
    booking, 66
    expectations, 68–69
    followup, 30
    living treatment plan, 104–106
    notes, 50
Aptensio, *see* methylphenidate
aripiprazole, 256
ashwagandha, 149
Ativan, *see* lorazepam
atomoxetine, 258
augment, 197, 202, 215, 247, 256
Aventyl, *see* nortriptyline

B12, *see* Vitamin B12
behavioural activation, 233
benzodiazepines, 192–194
    cognitive problems, 208

sleep, 207
withdrawal, 193
bibliotherapy, 234
binge-eating disorder, 16
biopsychosocial model, 10
Biphentin, *see* methylphenidate
bipolar disorder
   alcohol, 138
   antidepressants, 188
   cannabis, 140
   criteria, 178
   mood stabilizers, 194
   screening, 74
   sleep, 136
birth defect, *see* pregnancy
blood test, *see* laboratory test
borage, 149
borderline personality disorder, 18
brain fog, 135, *see also* cognitive problems, 182
brexpiprazole, 256
bulimia nervosa, 16, 133
bupropion, 186, 204, 245
   anxiety, 186
Buspar, *see* buspirone
buspirone, 205, 251

caffeine, 72, 136–137
   with l-theanine, 146
CAM, *see* complementary and alternative medicine
CAMH, 142
cancellation list, 66
CANMAT, *see* guidelines
cannabis, 139–142
carbamazepine, 253
CBD, *see* cannabis
CBT, 155, 156, 231–233
Celexa, *see* citalopram
chamomile, 149
choline, 146, 207
cholinergic, *see* anticholinergic
chronic illness, 11, 30
chronic illnesses, 47, 122
Cipralex, *see* escitalopram
citalopram, 241

client-centered therapy, 238
clinic, 47, 62, 68
   walk-in, 51
clomipramine, 247
clonazepam, 249
clonidine, 258
cognitive behavioural therapy, *see* CBT
cognitive distortions, 232
cognitive problems, xi, 19, 122, 186, 193, 199, 207, 208
   treatment, 128, 182
   treatments, 127
cognitive restructuring, 232
collaboration, 32, 100
collateral, 42
comorbid, 10, 19
complementary and alternative medicine, 143
compounding, 202, 215
comprehensive care, 3
concentration, *see* cognitive problems
Concerta, *see* methylphenidate
confirmation bias, 87
conspiracy, 175
constipation, 183, 209
consultation, *see* referral
cortisol, 130, 135, 137
cost, 23
   lab tests, 129
   physical illness, 123
   therapy, 157, 163–166
   treatment, 173
counselling, *see* therapy
counsellor, *see* therapist
credibility, 82
crisis, 14, 21, 37, 170, 171
   personality disorders, 18
   code word, 41
   resources, 38
cross-taper, 216
CT, *see* imaging
Cymbalta, *see* duloxetine
cyproheptadine, 205
cytochrome P450, 187

DBT, 155, 236–237
dementia, *see* cognitive problems
Depakote, *see* valproic acid
depression, 6, 10, 19, 133, 178, 188, 206, 208
    medication, 168, 177, 185
    risk, 121, 123, 125, 136, 141
    scales, 57
    side effect, 122
    treatment, 24, 127, 128, 130, 135, 142, 143, 147, 157, 175
desvenlafaxine, 243
Desyrel, *see* trazodone
Dexedrine, *see* amphetamine
DHEA, 130
diagnosis, 15–20, 57, 93
    differential, 17, 93
diagnostic overshadowing, 125
dialectical behavioural therapy, *see* DBT
diarrhea, 183, 209
diazepam, 249
diet, 133–135, 144, 206
dietary supplement, *see* natural health product
digestive, 134
digestive system, 187
doctor, 23, *see also* family doctor, psychiatrist
    ratings, 63
dopamine, 119
Dr. Google, 32, 81
Dr. Phil, 50
drugs, *see* illicit drugs
dry mouth, 207, 209
DSM, 16
duloxetine, 186, 244

EAP, 164
eating disorders, 16, 133
ECG, *see* electrocardiogram
eclectic therapy, 156
EEG, *see* electroenchephalogram
Effexor, *see* venlafaxine
Elavil, *see* amitriptyline

electrocardiogram, 131
electroencephalogram, 132
electronic medical records, *see* medical records
EMDR, 238
emergency room, 21, 38
emotional numbing, 182
employee assistance plan, *see* EAP
episodic care, 90, 107
Epival, *see* valproic acid
escitalopram, 242
estrogen, 130
eszopiclone, 250
evaluation, *see* treatment, evaluation
evidence, 82, 84–85, 113, 148, 152, 156, 160, 161
exercise, 135–136
existential psychotherapy, 238
expectations, 36
exposure, 232–233
Eye Movement Desensitization and Reprocessing, *see* EMDR

family
    communicating with, 40, 101
    medical appointments, 41
    meetings, 42
    support, 40
family doctor, 24
    advocate, 44
    communicating with, 49, 51, 88, 101
    gatekeeper, 45
    roles, 44
    without, 51
family history, 72
fatigue, 127, 128, 130, 137, 185, 202, 207
fax, 64
FDA, 83, 149, 239
ferritin, *see* iron
Fetzima, *see* levomilnacipran
fight-or-flight, 136, 154
fluoxetine, 241
fluvoxamine, 243
functioning, xi, 31, 170

GABA, 119, 145
gabapentin, 251
GAD-7, 57
gamma-aminobutyric acid, see GABA
gastrointestinal, see digestive system
general practitioner, see family doctor
genetics, 72, 169, 184, 188
Gestalt therapy, 238
gingko, 149, 205
goals, 93, 98, 101, 153, 157
Google, 81, see also Dr. Google
    Docs, 51
    Scholar, 87
grounding, 154, 236
group therapy, 23, 152–154, 166
guanfacine, 258
guidelines, 104, 184
    CANMAT, 157
    cannabis, 142
    nutritional, 144

hallucinogen, 142
headache, 183, 189, 209
Health Canada, 83, 149, 239
health insurance, 23, 37, 164
herbal, 147, see also natural health product
high-functioning, see functioning
history, 15, 36, 70–71
homelessness, 13
hormones, 130
hospital
    inpatient, 14, 24
    involuntary, 14, 174
    outpatient, 24, 62
humanistic therapy, 238
hypnotics, 191–194
hypomania, see bipolar disorder

illicit drugs, 142, 187, 189, 194, 199
imaging, 131
Imovane, see zopiclone
Inderal, see propranolol
inflammation, 125, 135

information overload, 46–47
inositol, 146
inpatient, see hospital
insomnia, 130, 136, 137, 141, 145, 146, 186, 192, 203, 207
interaction, 150, 169, 187, 267
interpersonal psychotherapy, see IPT
interventions, see treatments
interviews, 67–74
Intuniv, see guanfacine
involuntary commitment, see hospital
IPT, 235–236
iron, 127–128
irritability, 73, 130, 136, 193, 218

kava, 148
Klonopin, see clonazepam

l-theanine, 146
laboratory test, 15, 94, 127–132, 144, 195
Lamictal, see lamotrigine
lamotrigine, 254
Latuda, see lurasidone
lavender, 149
lemon balm, 149
levomilnacipran, 247
Lexapro, see escitalopram
lifestyle factors, 133–142, 175
lisdexamfetamine, see amphetamine
lithium, 252
living treatment plan, 89–108, 113, 157, 212
    example, 90
long-term disability, 164
lorazepam, 248
Lunesta, see eszopiclone
lurasidone, 256
Luvox, see fluvoxamine
Lyrica, see pregabalin

maca, 205
major depressive disorder, 157, see also depression
mania, see bipolar disorder
MAOI, 247

medical records, 36, 47
medications, 167–219
melatonin, 146
memory, *see* cognitive problems
menopause, 218
mental illness
    causes, 10
    criteria, 16
    definition, 9
    severity, xi, 12–13, 45
    understanding, 40
metabolism, *see* absorption
methylphenidate, 257
mindfulness, 154, 234
minerals, *see* vitamins
Minipress, *see* prazosin
mirtazapine, 186, 244
modafinil, 258
mood logs, 232
mood stabilizers, 194–197
mood swing, 122, 134, 136, 218
motivation, xi, 73, 171, 185, 188
MRI, *see* imaging

natural health product, 71, 83, 122, 143, 149, 150
nausea, 183, 186, 189, 209
neuroscience, 115–120
neurotransmitters, 119
nicotine, 138
nightmare, 141, 198, 200, 207
norepinephrine, 119
nortriptyline, 186, 246
notes, 35, 42, 50, 55, 105, 106
nutraceutical, *see* natural health product
nutrition, *see* diet

off-label, 229, 240
olanzapine, 255
Omega-3, 146
opioid, 142, 194
OTIS, 217
oxcarbazepine, 253

pain, 177, 186, 209
Paltrow, Gwyneth, 50

Pamelor, *see* nortriptyline
panic, 137, 154, 170, 193
parents, 41
paroxetine, 204, 241
passionflower, 149
patent extenders, 86
patient navigation, 30–31, 223
Paxil, *see* paroxetine
peer support, 22, 152, 153
perimenopause, 217
personality disorders, 17
pharmacist, 150, 174, 187, 203, 214
phenylalanine, 147
physical health, *see* physical illness
physical illness, 71, 121–126
physician, *see* medical doctor
poop-out, 128, 188, 216
postpartum, 217
posttraumatic stress disorder, *see* PTSD
prazosin, 252
predatory journals, 82
pregabalin, 251
pregnancy, 187, 216–217
prioritization, 45, 65
Pristiq, *see* desvenlafaxine
privacy laws, 37
problem-solving therapy, 235
progesterone, 130
prolactin, 130, 205, 255
propranolol, 252
Prozac, *see* fluoxetine
psychiatric survivor, 174
psychiatrist, 23, 24
psychiatry, 23, 24
psychodynamic therapy, 237
psychoeducation, 234
psychologist, 23
psychology, 23
psychosis, 122, 140, 197
psychotherapy, *see* therapy
PTSD, 73, 141, 238

QT prolongation, 131
quetiapine, 254

rating scales, 57–59, 104

receptor, 119
referral, 45, 61–66
    failures, 64
    letter, 63
regulated professionals, 161
relaxation, 235
Remeron, see mirtazapine
resilience, 171, 182, 224
restless legs, 127, 208
Rexulti, see brexpiprazole
rhodiola, 149
Risperdal, see risperidone
risperidone, 255
Ritalin, see methylphenidate
Rivotril, see clonazepam
roseroot, 149
rule out, 18, 93–95, 101

safety plan, 37
saffron, 149, 205
SAMe, 145
schizophrenia, 13, 170
secondary action, 186
sedatives, 191–194
self-harm, 37, 71
Seroquel, see quetiapine
serotonin, 119
    and exercise, 135
serotonin syndrome, 148, 189
sertraline, 242
severity, see symptoms, functioning, mental illness
sexual dysfunction, 183, 204–205, 215
side effects, 201–209
silver bullet, 39, 88, 113, 222
skullcap, 149
sleep, 136–137, 198
sleep apnea, 136, 194, 207
sleep hygiene, 136
sliding fee scale, 165
SMART goals, 94
social anxiety, 12, 138
social history, 73
social media, 82
somatic, 124

SSRI, 179, 205
St. John's wort, 147
Stevens-Johnson Syndrome, 254
stigma, viii, 18, 52
stimulants, 199
Strattera, see atomoxetine
Sublinox, see zolpidem
suicide, 37, 71
    antidepressants, 188
    bipolar disorder, 140
    doctor, 46
supplement, see natural health product
supportive psychotherapy, 237
sweating, 183, 189, 207
symptom mapping, 185
symptoms
    describing, 55
    frequency, 57
    impact, 57
    severity, 57, 104
    terminology, 56
synapse, 117
syndromes, 15
system failures, 2–3, 25–26

Tegretol, 253
testosterone, 130, 205
THC, see cannabis
therapist, 159–166
therapy, 151–166
thought records, 232
thyroid, 130
time pressure, 46
tobacco, 138
trauma, see PTSD
travel, 218
trazodone, 186, 250
treatment
    decisions, 6, 100, 102, 175
    evaluation, 104
    plan, 89, see also living treatment plan
treatments, 111–219
    new, 85
tremor, 128, 183, 189, 208

Trileptal, see oxcarbazepine
Trintellix, see vortioxetine
tryptophan, 145
turmeric, 149
tyrosine, 147

valerian, 149
validation, 83
Valium, see diazepam
valproic acid, 253
venlafaxine, 204, 243
Viibryd, see vilazodone
vilazodone, 247
Vitamin B12, 128–129, 135, 145
Vitamin D, 129
vitamins, 127–130, 134–135
vortioxetine, 247
Vyvanse, see amphetamine

weight, 133, 186, 196, 198, 205
Wellbutrin, see bupropion
withdrawal, 202, 204, 216
    alcohol, 139
    antidepressant, 183
    benzodiazepine, 192
    caffeine, 137
    mood stabilizer, 196
workbooks, 152, 166, 234
workplace, 37
worldview, 161

Xanax, see alprazolam

yohimbine, 205

z-drugs, 192
Zoloft, see sertraline
zolpidem, 249
zopiclone, 250
Zyprexa, see olanzapine

Acknowledgements

This book wouldn't exist without the collective wisdom, experience—and yes, pain, frustration, and disappointment—of hundreds of patients, their family members, and healthcare providers. Thanks to everyone who gave so generously of their time, freely sharing their stories of both good and bad experiences with mental health care.

Many people we talked to had been dealing with mental health challenges, their own or those of others, for years or decades. They weren't shy when sharing insights about what went well and what didn't. Most often, they talked about things they didn't know at the time or incorrect assumptions they'd made. "If I only knew then what I know now," they'd say, "things would have turned out a lot differently." Many commented that their mental health care was a tremendous learning experience, one they never thought they'd need to go through.

Some people scoff at the idea that patients benefit from knowing about certain aspects of their treatments and how the health system works behind the scenes. We beg to differ. The breadth of material covered in this book reflects the range of issues multiple people have directly struggled with. At the same time, it's easy to go overboard on the details. We appreciate everyone who helped us isolate and distill which parts are truly useful in practice.

We're grateful for those who provided feedback on early drafts of parts or all of the manuscript. They included Marla Abells-Segal, Carolyn Boutillier, Bev Cooke, Dr. Jon Davine, Bill Lysak, Evelyn Lysak, Tania Lysak, Dr. Michael Mawdsley, Ryan McDonald, Lauralee McDougall, Lindsay Millala, Kyle Parrott, Leanne Parrott, Dr. Laura Phillips, Lana Tong, and Christina Vesty. The final result is much tighter and more coherent for all your efforts.

Our editor, Peggy Herring, was a pleasure to work with. Her contributions shine through on every page. If errors crept in, they were doubtless a result of our compulsion to make "just one more" change after the fact. Sorry, Peggy. Hina Shakti was endlessly patient with our indecision around the cover design, providing us with numerous alternatives until we were finally happy.

Finally, thanks to everyone, especially current patients, who encouraged us, and shared ideas for book titles and cover concepts. Thanks for putting up with what must have seemed to be outlandish questions at times. We are grateful for those who graciously offered their time and talents.

Thanks for sharing the belief that your experiences with mental health care will make a positive difference in the lives of others.

About the Authors

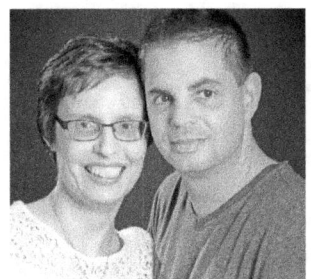

Dr. Pauline Lysak is an accomplished general psychiatrist, with a particular interest in treating complex patients having both physical and mental illnesses. Dr. Lysak obtained her medical degree with honors in research at the University of Alberta. She completed her psychiatry residency at McMaster University. She subsequently completed the prestigious Advanced Health Leadership Executive Program at the Rotman School of Management. She has practiced and held leadership positions in a cancer centre's psycho-oncology service, a program for complex psychiatric patients at a nationally renowned mental health and addiction facility, and in several hospital-based and private outpatient practices.

Mark Roseman is a software developer, entrepreneur, writer, and mental health advocate. He previously worked and published extensively on topics related to user experience and technology to support collaboration between groups of people. He also founded two software startup companies. More recently, he has been supporting Pauline with her psychiatry practice.

They live in Victoria, BC, Canada. You can contact them via mhnav.com.

www.ingramcontent.com/pod-product-compliance
Lightning Source LLC
Chambersburg PA
CBHW071231070526
44583CB00017B/2135